DATE DUE

DEMCO

Living With Myasthenia Gravis

Living With Myasthenia Gravis
A Bright New Tomorrow

By

JEAN WELCH KEMPTON

With Forewords by

William H. Everts, M.D., Med. Sc. D. (D-PN)

and

William M. McKinney, M.D.

Illustrations by Joseph Roselli

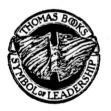

CHARLES C THOMAS · PUBLISHER
Springfield · Illinois · U. S. A.

Published and Distributed Throughout the World by
CHARLES C THOMAS • PUBLISHER
BANNERSTONE HOUSE
301–327 East Lawrence Avenue, Springfield, Illinois, U. S. A.
NATCHEZ PLANTATION HOUSE
735 North Atlantic Boulevard, Fort Lauderdale, Florida, U. S. A.

With THOMAS BOOKS *careful attention is given to all details of
manufacturing and design. It is the Publisher's desire to present books
that are satisfactory as to their physical qualities and artistic possibilities
and appropriate for their particular use. THOMAS BOOKS will be true
to those laws of quality that assure a good name and good will.*

Printed in the United States of America
K-3

To my family, in gratitude for their care and devotion.

To Herb Sander, a myasthenic, who gave courage and hope to so many other myasthenics.

To all myasthenics and the physicians and scientists working to find a cure.

Foreword

THE AUTHOR of this book is uniquely qualified to suggest practical ideas for a "bright new tomorrow." She has personally experienced many of the problems and has actively researched workable solutions for patients with myasthenia gravis. Her insight and dedication to the problem are evident in the manuscript. I believe that this book will have great value to patients with myasthenia, their families, physicians and students, as well as other people associated with myasthenia gravis. The synthesis of medical knowledge with practical application will make this a most interesting and informative contribution.

WILLIAM M. McKINNEY
Associate Professor
Department of Neurology
The Bowman Gray School of Medicine
Winston-Salem, North Carolina

Foreword

I T is a real pleasure to acknowledge this book which has been over thirty-five years in the making. Early in 1935, at the Neurological Institute of New York, Miss Jean-Louise Welch, a young Cornell University student, was admitted critically ill with what we know as myasthenia gravis. The opportunity was thus afforded to carry out intensive clinical research on this very disabling disorder. After much study of the then known biochemistry of the nervous system and the role of acetylcholine and pharmacology of physostigmine, all was ready to use the drug physostigmine in an effort to combat this disease. Then perchance, the new drug prostigmin became available and was thus used instead, with the dramatic response described so aptly by the recipient, the author of this manuscript. Other drugs such as ephedrine and potassium chloride were also used and were variably effective.

The keystone of therapy was thus prostigmin which was then carefully titrated orally and brought out in tablet form as reported in the basic research, December 1935, in the Bulletin of the Neurological Institute of New York. The following year a full course of x-ray therapy to the thymus gland was administered because of a suggested enlargement of the thymus shadows in the x-rays of her chest and the possible relationship to myasthenia gravis. Evaluation of the effectiveness of this treatment was difficult to qualify, for our patient continued to sustain herself well and show continued improvement.

During this time and the years that followed, there were of course many new patients with many variations of the myasthenic disorder examined and treated with varying success. The author came to know and to study some of these patients and compare their individual reactions and responses, not only relative to their medication but their living adaptations, dietary habits, and psychological outlook. Being a young woman of very fine mind and collegiate training, she was encouraged to ever explore her own and others' health adjustments and the symptomatic peregrinations of this subtle disabling disorder. She displayed in the very best manner the courage to endure and the determination to make the best of it at all times.

Long ago, then, a book for understanding and a guide to living was in formation in the mind of our author. This book, presented in clear and simple language, should prove very helpful and instill a brighter outlook for the future in all myasthenic patients and their families and be assistive to the practicing physician who is called upon to care for patients with this disorder. The author, essentially symptom-free and the picture of good health today, continues her dedicated, very busy, interesting life, and her presentation here is an inspiring record of accomplishment.

WILLIAM H. EVERTS

Preface

ℙℙℙℙℙℙℙℙℙℙℙℙℙℙℙℙℙℙℙℙℙℙℙℙℙℙℙℙℙℙℙℙℙℙℙℙℙℙℙ

Living With Myasthenia Gravis has developed from nearly forty years of experience as a myasthenic. Starting as an active teenager, I have gone through the throes of having a very advanced case during a time when the disease was considered hopeless to becoming an extremely active middle-aged woman in remission.

The symptoms developed slowly and the disease went unrecognized until I was in a very advanced stage. I was sent to the Neurological Institute of the Columbia-Presbyterian Medical Center in New York City. Because there was no hope for me and death was imminent, my mother wanted me home to die.

While waiting in a wheelchair to be discharged, I stopped breathing. A nurse happened to come by just then to say goodbye. When she couldn't get my pulse she ran for help.

It was fortunate that a group of doctors were making rounds then. All came hurrying and drastic measures were taken. A young resident neurologist, Dr. William Everts, was one of the doctors. He pulled me through the night and vowed that because of my youth he would find something to relieve my suffering. He spent all of his free time in the library studying, searching for some clue, some medicine, some hope for this baffling, devastating disease.

It looked for a while as though Dr. Everts's search would be in vain for death started to overtake me several times. It is a curious feeling to hear a chaplain pray for your departing soul and your family discuss funeral arrangements. It was considered impossible for me to live. Once my death certificate was made out ready for signature.

The historic day that the young neurologist decided to try an injection of Prostigmin® will be imprinted on my mind forever. I was as helpless as a rag doll, unable to lift my head from the pillow without assistance. I saw through slits as both eyelids drooped so badly. My speech was extremely weak and slurred. There was constant danger of my choking to death as I could scarcely swallow. It took me an hour to choke down an eggnog. Breathing was an effort and I had not been out of bed for three months.

After the injection of Prostigmin, in just a minute my breathing became deeper. My masked expression began to melt like paraffin under heat. My eyelids opened and my voice became clear and strong. In five minutes I sat up alone and excitedly looked at myself in the mirror which my doctor extended. He wanted to know if I looked like my real self. What a thrill for both of us to have the horrible symptoms of myasthenia gravis disappear like magic. I remember asking, "What have you given me? What has happened?"

The doctor gaily picked up the hypodermic syringe and waved it. "Black Magic," he replied. It truly seemed like magic for in just twelve minutes I got out of bed and walked the length of the corridor as normally as anyone. In a short time my tray came and I sat in a chair beside my bed and ate with great relish the first normal meal I had eaten in about two years. No meal since has ever tasted quite as good.

Just as magically as the symptoms disappeared, they reappeared, only this time I knew they would not be permanent. Since, at that time, I was the first person in America to have had the drug used to relieve myasthenia gravis, no one knew how often it could be given, how the side effects would be tolerated or what the accumulative effect would be.

Then began a long period of work and experimentation by the doctors and the laboratories that made the drug. I was given the privilege of being included as part of the team and participated in the development of first a liquid and then the pill form which is now used all over the world. In December 1935 Dr. Everts published his early researches, including my case history, under the title: The Treatment of Myasthenia Gravis by the Oral Administration of Prostigmin. It appeared in the *Bulletin of the Neurological Institute of New York* (vol. iv). Dr. Everts has continued to be my guiding and ever encouraging physician over these many years. To him I owe my life.

It is with a background of personal experience with all of the dangers, problems, frustrations, discouragements and tribulations a myasthenic endures, the trial of various medications and a great deal of research, that I have prepared this manuscript. It is not only for the myasthenic but also for all of the various disciplines that surround them—physicians, nurses, dentists, ministers, social workers, psychologists and psychiatrists, parents, husbands, wives, sweethearts and friends. My earnest prayer is that through this means, understanding, hope and courage can be given to the one who is ill with myasthenia gravis.

JEAN WELCH KEMPTON

Acknowledgments

━━

THIS BOOK is the result of the concerted effort of a number of people. I am especially indebted to Dr. William M. McKinney, Assistant Professor of Neurology of The Bowman Gray School of Medicine, Winston Salem, North Carolina. He gave so generously of his time in supervising the details, guiding my efforts and in arranging for me to use the facilities of The Bowman Gray School of Medicine. It was through Dr. McKinney's efforts that I received a small grant to cover the expenses of preparing the manuscript from The Mary E. Welch Myasthenia Gravis Research Fund.

Other persons at The Bowman Gray School of Medicine gave valuable assistance. Dr. William McLean was consultant on the chapter on childhood myasthenia. Mrs. Erika Love, Chief Librarian, gave technical assistance and encouragement. Mr. George Lynch, Director of Audiovisual Resources, supervised the illustrations and Miss Louise MacMillan, Assistant Editor of *The North Carolina Medical Journal,* was editorial consultant.

In addition, I appreciate the encouragement and assistance given by Dr. William H. Everts, Florida neurologist; Mr. Donald Kempton, psychologist, who served as consultant on the psychological aspects of the book; and Miss Mary McAllister, a young adult who has battled multiple handicaps, for her advice on the youth section.

I am grateful to Dr. J. E. Hebeler, Assistant Professor of Pediatrics, University of Texas, Medical Branch, for suggesting the chapters on childhood myasthenia and tips for teenagers; Adelle Davis, nutritionist and author, who generously shared her research on myasthenia gravis; and Dr. Woodward Farmer, internist, for his helpful comments after reviewing the manuscript.

Mrs. Jane Ellsworth, mother of a myasthenic and founder of The Myasthenia Gravis Foundation, Inc., kindly reviewed the manuscript and gave helpful suggestions. I also appreciate the time taken by members of the Medical Advisory Board of the Myasthenia Gravis Foundation, Inc., who reviewed the manuscript.

A number of patients and relatives of patients were asked to review the manuscript and to answer two questionnaires pertaining to it. I appreciate their efforts and helpful comments. The patients were Mrs. Lavonia Gore, North Carolina; Miss Jennie Sindin, Pennsylvania; Mrs. Leo Weinerb, Pennsylvania; and Mrs. Dorothy Parney, Pennsylvania. Relatives of myasthenics included Mrs. Howard Welch, North Carolina; Mrs. Louis Harfin, Long Island; Mrs. Dorothy Stone, New York; and Mrs. Mahlon Adams, North Carolina.

To all of these wonderful people and to the many unnamed ones who were an inspiration and a help, I give my deepest gratitude. Jointly we hope our efforts will provide help and encouragement to myasthenics and their families and to all those working with the disease to whom our efforts have been directed.

J. W. K.

SO MANY HEARTS ARE BRAVE

by Grace Noll Crowell

So many hearts are brave. Each day I see
The lifted banners of their courage shine
Out of the myriad eyes that look in mine:

The banners mankind carry as they march
To prove that they are undefeated still,
Though tired feet must often drag behind;
Though there be scarcely strength to climb the hill,
Brave women and brave men, who go their way
Without blare of music down the street;
Without cheers, or the encouragement
Of words that would be heartening and sweet.

So many hearts have the courage to go on
Undaunted by their loss, or pain, or fear;
Beaten perhaps, yet holding in their souls
The beautiful bright quality of cheer.
So many hearts are brave—though well they know
How rough the road is that their feet must go.

Contents

Living With Myasthenia Gravis

There is a limit to health: Disease is
always a near neighbor.
AESCHYLUS: Agamemnon
c. 490 B. C.

Disease is very old and nothing
about it has changed. It is we who
change as we learn to recognize what
was formerly imperceptible.
J. M. CHARCOT
De l'expectation in Medicine
1957.

1

The Disease

❥❥❥❥❥❥❥❥❥❥❥❥❥❥❥❥❥❥❥❥❥❥❥❥❥❥❥❥❥❥❥❥❥

So you have myasthenia gravis! It may comfort you to know
that you are not alone. It is estimated that there are from
30,000 to nearly a million myasthenics in the United States. It is
believed that for every diagnosed case there are many more un-
diagnosed ones. As more doctors become familiar with the disease,
more cases are properly diagnosed.

Today your chances of recovery are 80 to 90 percent. Thirty-
five years ago they were only five percent. Never has so much
time, effort and money been concentrated on finding the cause
and cure. Doctors and biochemists all over the world are writing
of the promising progress which is being made in the study of
this disease and its cause.

What is myasthenia gravis? It is just what the name means.
Mys is Greek for muscle and *asthenia* means weakness. *Gravis*
is, of course, Latin for very serious or grave. However, one does
not have to be in a seriously weakened condition to have myasthenia gravis. Today, many discovered cases are very mild because of early diagnosis made possible by special tests.

What causes this strange muscle disease? That is still a mystery.
It seems that something goes wrong with your chemistry which

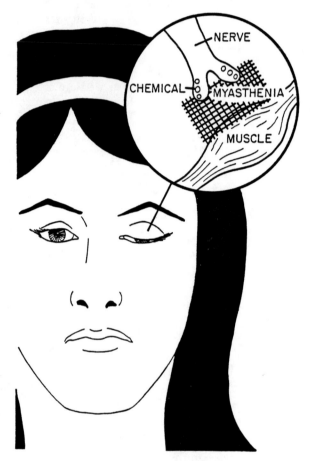

The Chemical Breakdown

causes what amounts to an "electrical short circuit." It is believed that there is a failure in the electrical stimulus which carries the impulse from the brain to the nerve which in turn makes the muscle move. In other words, you are loaded with a mammoth telegraph system which constantly sends messages to the central office—your brain. In your case, something happens to prevent the message from getting through or else it only goes through weakly.

The impulse passes over many little bridges or "synapse" points to carry out reflex or involuntary acts. It is at these little bridges or reflex points that the myasthenia patient suffers. The chemistry is disturbed so that the nerve impulses are interfered with and will not pass in proper or in sufficient manner so that muscle movement is either weakened or impossible.

Suppose you have weakness in your hands. You will be able to open and close them in rapid succession only for a few times. It will become increasingly difficult for you until you cannot open or close your hand at all. The impulse goes through the first few times but then fails to pass over the bridge in sufficient strength to open or close your hand. After a few minutes of rest, you again can open and close your hand. The impulse has been restored. Of course, this is oversimplification. If you want to get really technical, a review of the literature will give a variety of descriptions. We shall explore a few of them.

Although myasthenia gravis is a little known disease, it is not a new one. As early as 1672, Thomas Willis, an English doctor, wrote about myasthenia gravis. His paper had the imposing title of *Discourses Concerning the Soul of Brutes*. He described the patients as

> . . . those laboring with want of spirits who will exercise local motions, as well as they can, in the early morning are able to walk firmly, to fling about their arms . . . hither and thither, or take up heavy things; before noon the stock of spirits, which had flowed into the muscles, they are scarce able to move hand or foot.

He goes on to give a case study of a patient whom he describes as

> . . . a prudent honest woman who for many years hath been obnoxious to this spurious palsie not only in her members, but also in her tongue; she for some time can speak freely and readily enough, but after she spoke long or hastily, or eagerly, she is not able to speak a word, but becomes mute as a fish, nor can she recover the use under an hour or two.

Until 1927 only three hundred cases were reported. It was considered a rare and baffling disease. Although still baffling, rapid diagnostic tests and better-informed doctors can now recognize the disease and have brought to light many new cases. It is no

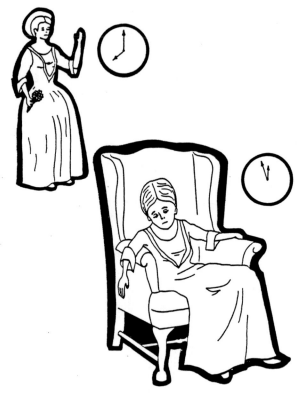

First Reported Case

longer considered rare. Today, hundreds of cases of myasthenia gravis are being studied at various medical centers throughout the United States and the rest of the world.

It seems to be agreed that there are four distinct forms of myasthenia gravis. Two involve babies and children and two involve only adults. A myasthenic mother can transmit symptoms to her baby. These symptoms show up at birth and then disappear. Then there is the type that develops some time during childhood. It affects both sides of the body equally, such as both hands or both legs. In these cases, the mother is not a myasthenic but there frequently are cases of it in the family.

Of the two adult forms of myasthenia gravis, the most common one can vary between a mild type which can affect a single group of muscles, such as an eyelid, to a severe form which affects the total body. In many of these there is an enlargement of the thymus and there may even be a tumor on the thymus. The second type is most unusual. It is the only one in which a muscle atrophy may develop.

The symptoms of myasthenia gravis seem to vary with each patient. One may have one or all of a variety of symptoms. There may be heaviness in the legs, fatigue upon the slightest exertion, drooping of the eyelid in one or both eyes, double vision, difficulty in swallowing and chewing, sagging jaws, or a masked expression. The voice may weaken until it is inaudible and the speech is slurred. There may be weakness of the cardiac muscles

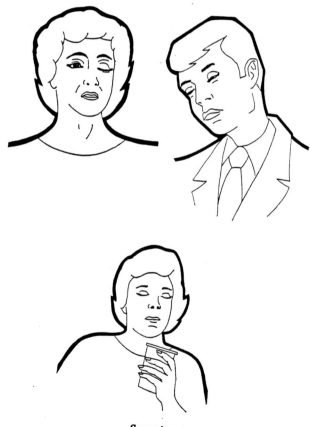

Symptoms

which may cause palpitation and an abnormally rapid heart action. There can be weakness of the trunk and upper and lower limbs. The neck muscles may be so weak the head bobs like a rag doll's unless supported.

It is characteristic of myasthenia gravis that as the day wears on you will become increasingly weaker. You generally feel your best in the morning. You feel better after periods of rest. On some days you will feel worse than on others. There will be some days when you may feel quite well. Some people even experience periods of months or years when they feel well. These are called remissions. A remission sometimes ends very suddenly for no apparent reason. This is part of the mystery which surrounds the disease. Weakness can be increased by overactivity, the menses, respiratory infections and emotional upsets.

The cause of myasthenia gravis is still unknown. There are, however, several theories. The most popular one is based on the belief that there is a defect in the neuromuscular transmission which appears to be due to a competitive-type block which inhibits the motor end plate depolarizing action of acetylcholine released from the motor nerve endings. In other words, in order to transmit the message or impulse from the nerve to the muscle, a chemical known as acetylcholine must be in proper balance with an enzyme, cholinesterase. When this does not happen, there is a block at the muscle-nerve junction which prevents the movement of the muscle.

Some doctors theorize that myasthenia gravis is caused by a dysfunction of the endocrine system. An early scientist felt that the dysfunction of either the adrenals or parathyroids caused disturbances of the sympathetic nervous system which disordered the blood supply to the muscle. This resulted in the exhaustion and the abnormal electrical responses at the motor end plates. A relationship to the thyroid gland has also received attention.

From the 1930's on, much attention was directed toward the thymus gland. It was found that a large percentage of myasthenics have enlarged thymus glands. This gland is found in the chest behind the upper end of the breastbone. Normally in an infant the gland is large and helps to produce antibodies against infections. The gland normally shrinks at puberty but for some un-

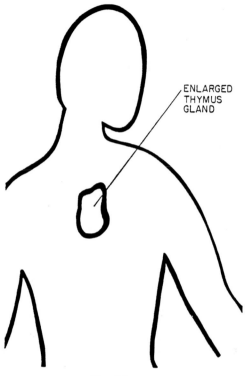

ENLARGED
THYMUS
GLAND

The Thymus

known reason this does not happen in many myasthenics. Their thymus glands remain large.

For many years the removal of the thymus gland, either by surgery or by deep x-ray, was advised for myasthenics with enlarged thymus glands who had generalized symptoms. It was found that young women in their twenties showed the best improvement. Many lost all of their myasthenic symptoms. For some unknown reason, men seldom showed improvement.

Because antibodies against the voluntary muscles can be found in the blood serum of some myasthenics, it is now thought by some that the disease is an autoimmune disorder. Abnormal cells have been found in lymph nodes, the spleen and the thymus, as well as in the tonsils. The body, it seems, reacts to the abnormal cells by building antibodies just like it does for a foreign substance. The body then retains various amounts of the antibodies at the junction of the nerve and muscle. In other words, the myasthenic becomes allergic to himself, to his own antigens. Recent studies suggest the possibility that one function of the thymus is to combat bacterial infections. It is believed to be the first organ to develop antibodies.

Muscle weakness has been developed experimentally in a rabbit's ear using the autoimmunity theory. The weakness was reversed by the same drugs given for myasthenia gravis. To be able to reproduce a myasthenic-like weakness in a laboratory animal is a major research advance. New drugs can then be tested without endangering the patient.

Another new technique has been perfected which also will be a helpful tool in the development of new treatments. A way has been found to keep alive a half inch of rib muscle taken from a myasthenic. This enables further study of muscle reactions and the reactions of various chemicals on the muscle without hurting the patient.

There is some evidence that myasthenia gravis has some effect on menstruation, pregnancy and menopause. For this reason some investigators have been exploring the possible role the sex glands might play in the disease. So far, no definite conclusions have been reached.

Another group of investigators are working on the theory that myasthenia gravis is a metabolic disorder. They feel that the neuromuscular block is caused by some breakdown in protein-enzyme metabolism. Some have likened the disease to a nutritional deficiency and have obtained good results through using nutrition therapy.

There are others who have pioneered in experiments which appear to demonstrate that the disease could be of a bacterial origin due to the presence of cocci in and between the muscle fibers. It is believed that these bacteria may give off a toxin which could cause muscle fatigue. One study shows that 35 percent of twenty patients had more or less severe infections in the upper respiratory tract just prior to the development of myasthenia gravis.

If you feel confused at this point, it is no wonder, but out of confusion can come order. In *Letters and Social Aims*, Ralph Waldo Emerson said, "Our knowledge is the amassed thought and experience of innumerable minds." It was only thirty-five years ago that Prostigmin revolutionized the treatment of myasthenia gravis and took the hopelessness out of it. Since that time much knowledge about the disease has been amassed by some of the greatest scientists in the world. Who knows? Maybe tomorrow, next week, next month or next year, the complete cure will be found!

2

How It Is Treated

✛✛✛✛✛✛✛✛✛✛✛✛✛✛✛✛✛✛✛✛✛✛✛✛✛✛✛✛✛✛✛✛✛✛

SINCE myasthenia gravis was recognized, its treatment has gone through various cycles. Early physicians, working on the theory that muscular contractions could be improved by increasing the creatine content of the muscle, fed their patients glycine or arginine. Although some benefit was shown in a few cases, the treatment proved to be a disappointment.

Up to 1930 treatment was generally restricted to rest, large doses of strychnine, sometimes arsenic, thyroid extract, parathyroid preparations, calcium and thorium were used. Most of the emphasis, however, was on complete rest.

Dr. Harriet Edgeworth accidentally found a new treatment in 1930. She had hay fever as well as myasthenia gravis. In an effort to find relief from hay fever, Dr. Edgeworth took ephedrine sulphate. She was surprised to note that the myasthenic symptoms also improved. Thus ephedrine sulphate became an accepted treatment. It is still used by some today to supplement one of the new anticholinesterase medications.

The real turning point came in England in 1934 when Dr. Mary Walker noted that the symptoms of myasthenia gravis and curare poisoning were similar. Since physostigmine would unblock the

12

adverse effect of curare, Dr. Walker gave physostigmine to a patient with myasthenia gravis. The patient lost all of his symptoms in a matter of minutes.

Physostigmine inactivates cholinesterase, prolonging and intensifying the action of acetylcholine. It improves the tone and action of skeletal muscles. However, it was found that too much physostigmine might also cause weakness as a side effect. This has been termed a crisis due to drug therapy. The discovery of physostigmine opened the door to the development of many other closely related drugs.

Prostigmin (Hoffman-La Roche), similar to physostigmine but without the many side effects, was first used in America in 1935 when it was given to a critically ill myasthenic when all other known treatments had failed. The improvement in the patient was rapid and dramatic.

Because the effectiveness of Prostigmin wore off in a few hours, repeated injections were necessary. It left the patient in a plight similar to a diabetic who has to take repeated doses of insulin. Not satisfied with the dependence of a patient upon multiple injections, Dr. William Everts worked with the laboratories that produced the drug to perfect a workable oral form. Oral Prostigmin, or Prostigmin Bromide as it was called, really emancipated the myasthenic. No longer was it a hopeless disease. It could be treated easily and effectively without a patient being dependent upon frequent hypodermic injections.

The next big step was the use of Prostigmin for a diagnostic test. It was found that only myasthenia gravis responds so dramatically to Prostigmin. If a patient is relieved of the symptoms by an injection of Prostigmin, a positive diagnosis can be made. This early diagnosis makes prompt treatment possible. The more serious aspects of the disease can then be minimized.

In 1952 an even faster diagnostic test, using a different drug, Tensilon,® was developed by Dr. Kermit Osserman. This is injected into the vein and takes only two minutes to strengthen muscles, whereas Prostigmin took several minutes. Tensilon also can be used to determine whether a crises is caused by overdosage or underdosage. It is curious that either too much or too little medicine can cause a serious reaction. The fact that Tensilon can determine the kind of reaction is lifesaving, since it indicates to the physician how much drug should be used.

Potassium chloride, which was used as early as 1935, is sometimes helpful in relieving myasthenic symptoms. If given in repeated small doses before the effect of Prostigmin wears off, the feeling of exhaustion is relieved and the improvement brought on by the drug is prolonged.

Because the effectiveness of Prostigmin is of short duration, in some cases of severe myasthenia gravis, massive doses have to be taken within a 24-hour period. A search for a longer-acting medication led to the development of Mestinon® (Hoffman-La Roche). This is an analogue of Prostigmin. Although Mestinon is slower acting, it sometimes has a longer effectiveness.

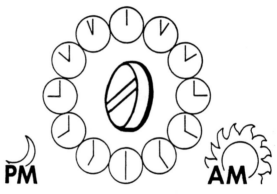

Time-Span Pills

Time-span tablets of both Prostigmin and Mestinon are a boon to severe myasthenics. These prolonged action tablets have three different layers of medication which become effective at various intervals. Time-span pills generally last two and a half times as long as regular pills. They are especially helpful in keeping a patient comfortable all night.

Mytelase® (Winthrop) is still another analogue of Prostigmin. It is reported to work better and to last longer than Mestinon. Some patients find fewer side effects. Some claim it causes less bronchial secretion than either Prostigmin or Mestinon. This can be a big advantage in some situations. Since Mytelase is combined with chloride instead of bromide, it can be used for patients who are sensitive to the bromide drugs.

These three drugs—Prostigmin, Mestinon and Mytelase—either alone or in combination, now constitute the most popular treatments for myasthenia gravis. It is important to recognize that each medication needs to be adjusted to meet the patient's particular needs. This may vary with the course of the illness.

Scientists in Vienna have altered the Prostigmin and Mestinon molecules and formed five other drugs similar to the parent drugs. They have a much stronger and longer-lasting action. These are

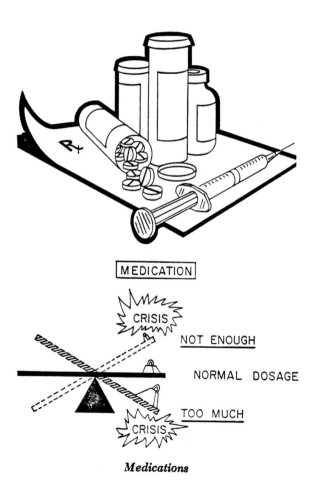

MEDICATION

CRISIS

NOT ENOUGH

NORMAL DOSAGE

TOO MUCH

CRISIS

Medications

still in the testing stage and only time and experience will prove their value.

A variety of other drugs have been and are being tested. WIN is one of these. It looked promising for a while but did not stand the test of time. A group of alkyl phosphates with long imposing names shortened to DFP, TEPP, HETP and OMPA were developed. Although they were useful, the side reactions prevented further investigation. Two others, PAM and DAM, were modified a bit with the hope that they would produce less side reactions. They also have not been generally accepted. Lycoramine, a derivative of galanthamine and germine diacetate, are being tried, with satisfactory results, by some doctors on selected patients. These may prove a welcome answer to many. There is still another drug which has shown promising results in the laboratory. It has not even been named but is known as IMK565.

When the adrenocorticotropic hormones (ACTH) were introduced, some physicians, working on the endocrine theory, thought this was going to be the answer. A few good results were reported, but here again there were many serious side reactions. ACTH is still used in those patients who fail to respond to the usual drugs, but it must be administered in a hospital with intensive care facilities and by a physician well experienced in the care of myasthenia gravis. The myasthenia weakness may increase while under treatment before the patient gets better.

Alternate-day high doses of prednisone, a corticosteroid, has been reported successful in a few patients.

From Russia and Germany come glowing reports of new drugs being tested there. Argentine doctors are using an operation on the carotid sinus which opens still another avenue of investigation. French medical journals also report on the operation which is thought to make the remaining nerves more sensitive to the action of certain body chemicals.

Most investigators insist there is no connection between myasthenia gravis and nutritional deficiency. Some, however, see a similarity. Doctors who have been treating myasthenia gravis with massive doses of certain vitamins report good results and have patients who have been in complete remission for a number of years. They use large doses of vitamin C, E, and B complex and a high-protein diet. Raw sugars and carbohydrates are kept low to reduce the tendency to puffiness and water retention.

The removal of the thymus gland, either by surgery or by treating with radiological therapy, is still being used in some cases. It is used primarily in severe cases among young women. Some thymus glands may have malignant tumors on them. There have been some cases of remissions following a thymectomy. This is especially true in young women.

Although a cure has not been found, so much work is being done in research laboratories and clinics all over the world, the solution is bound to be found. While these investigations in many different areas are being conducted, you can be kept comfortable and reasonably active. Patience and hope are very important ingredients of your treatment plus faith that a cure will be found. These should be taken in massive doses. Thomas Aquinas, back in 1265, said, "Faith has to do with things that are not seen, and hope with things that are not in hand."

3

How To Live With Illness

+O+O+O+O+O+O+O+O+O+O+O+O+O+O+O+O+O+O+O+O+O+O+O+O+O+O+O+O+O+O+O

O FTEN the test of courage is not to die but to live," said Alfieri
in *Orestes*. It does take a lot of courage to accept what cannot be changed, to see the challenge in revamping a way of life,
to establish a new set of goals and to find a new sphere in which
to work or play.

If you are one of the fortunate ones who have received early
diagnosis and are able to maintain normal activity on your medicine, wonderful. All you have to do is to take your medicine as
needed and avoid excessive fatigue and virus infections. You can
then go on your merry way as always.

If you are one of the majority, you are a little dizzy from the
merry-go-round of doctors you have seen. You have been from
internist to ophthalmologist, to psychiatrist, to neurologist. Your
head is spinning from the variety of diagnoses given. You no doubt
have taken the Tensilon test which established the fact that you
do have myasthenia gravis.

Now you need to accept the diagnosis and to adjust your life
accordingly. This is easier to say than to do but it is of prime
importance. If you choose to run the show your way, to ignore
warning signals, to take your medicine on a hit-or-miss schedule,
to consistently push yourself too hard, to ignore the precautions

18

given by the doctor and to think you can force your muscles to function when they are fatigued, then you are in for defeat.

If your case is acute, the doctor probably will want to hospitalize you until your medicine is stabilized. He may want you to stay in bed at home for a while, or he may want to restrict some of your activities to fit your limitations. Treatment will depend upon your symptoms and the severity of your illness. In any case, it is up to you to cooperate. There is an old Italian proverb: "Illness tells us what we are."

Most people fill their lives so full of activity they need jet propulsion to take them from one appointment to another. It is no wonder the human body cries out in protest. Some people fill their days with activities to avoid being alone with themselves. It is surprising to note the number of people who have to be constantly in the company of others, seeking praise and adulation in order to feel worthy of living. Others are just swept up in the momentum of this atomic era. They rush from this to that merely because everyone else is rushing.

There once was a man who so organized his time that every minute was used. He even read while walking. One day he met a friend who stopped him for a few minutes of conversation. When they parted, the man with the book suddenly stopped and called to his friend, "Say, was I coming or going?"

Many are not sure of the direction in which they are headed. Now, however, you are going to have time to learn to live with yourself and to find your direction.

In the first place, what are the things in life which are most important? Some psychologists say man has five basic drives: to be alive, to belong, to love and be loved, to believe in something greater than himself, and to excel in something. Myasthenia gravis is not going to prevent you from developing all of these drives.

You are alive. You belong to a family, a circle of friends, a community, a church or temple. You can love and be loved. You can believe in a Power greater than yourself and there are many things in which you can excel. You may not be able to swim the English channel or be a football hero but you can do a little re-evaluating and set goals that are within your reach.

Suppose, for instance, you were a young mother like Joan, with two children, the younger three and the older ten. The world did not come tumbling down because Joan had to spend some time in bed. On the contrary, it became an enriching experience for the whole family.

Joan had always been so busy she had little time to listen to the children. Now she had the sympathetic ear the children wanted and needed. A closer relationship and depth of understanding developed between them.

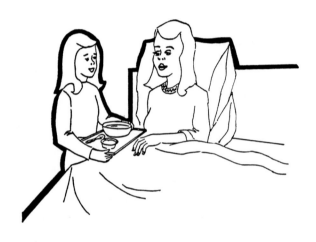

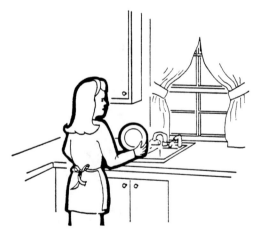

Children Can Help

Joan found that the three-year-old began to take great pride in doing things for herself. She learned to help set the table and to make her own bed. The ten-year-old learned to do simple ironing and cooking. Both of the children gained a new feeling of importance and achievement which greatly increased their self-confidence and independence.

It was a welcome change for Joan's husband to stay home from meetings and either read aloud to Joan after the children were in bed or play gin rummy. The more important role he had to play in the family seemed to improve his stature as a man.

You may be like John. To you comes the responsibility of earning the living to support your wife and children. Of course, it is hard to stop working for a while, but there is no need to push the panic button. Business concerns have insurance for just such emergencies. Surely you can get a leave-of-absence for enough time to again get your feet on the ground. You may need only to be transferred to a lighter job.

John was able to go back to work after a few months and to continue working until he was eligible for an early retirement. Then, because commuting to the city was a struggle for him, John retired and started an insurance business in his home.

Of course, the pension of an early retirement is not sufficient for you to belong to the country club, to take cruises or to send the children to college. Your wife may want to supplement the income. Is this so terrible? Over half of the married women are working now. It will not hurt the children to earn their own little expenses. They will come to value money more and the things they can have. The important thing is not how much of an income you have or who earns it, but the kind of family relationships you have and your attitudes toward each other.

Or, suppose you are a sweet young thing like Diane. She was a student in college, eager to grab life by the tail and give it a whirl, when myasthenia gravis hit her and hit her hard. She had to give up college and change her whole career plan. As soon as Diane was well enough, she ran a mail order gift and magazine business at home. Later, when medication gave her enough strength, she was able to secure an office position.

It is not the amount of trouble that comes into your life that

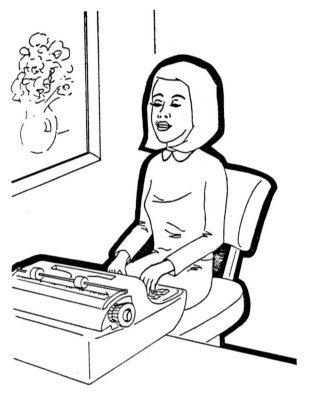

Patient Now a Typist

throws you into a tailspin. It is your attitude toward your problem that does. Everyone, strong or weak, goes through many crises throughout life. They must be faced. You cannot run away from them. There is an old Chinese proverb which says, "You cannot run away from trouble. Trouble runs faster than you."

A myasthenic must accept the fact that he has a puzzling disease that may suddenly leave of its own accord only to return just as suddenly. It may be that you never will be free of symptoms in spite of all you do. Medication may keep you comfortable and may prevent the more serious stages if you catch it early. On the other hand, you may be one of those who has disturbing reactions until the medicine best suited is found.

It will be up to you to design a way of living to fit your particular needs. You will need to separate the important from the unimportant. If you are used to being part of an active noisy crowd it will be hard for you to assume a more passive role. This is when you will come face to face with yourself and discover the kind of person you really are.

You may need to develop some inner resources. No matter how robust a person is or how self-sufficient he may be, no man lives completely alone. A crisis or illness often points this up and reveals depths of resources available, the love of another, the love

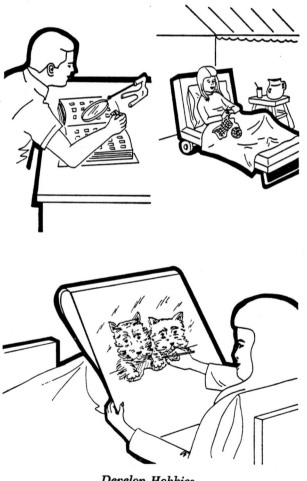

Develop Hobbies

of God. Of course, you must open your heart and mind to be receptive to these resources.

How long has it been since you have noticed the beauty of a sunset; listened to the melodic song of a thrush at twilight; or watched the changing patterns on the sidewalk made by sunlight dancing through the leaves? When did you last read a good, inspiring book?

Now is a good time to develop a hobby if you do not have one. Almost everyone wishes he had time to listen to records, to collect stamps, to watch birds, to label various collections, to raise African violets or to knit. Become absorbed in some interesting project.

One myasthenic began collecting dolls which led her to designing them professionally. She also studied the history of dolls and could trace civilization through them. When her speech became normal, she was a frequent speaker at schools, women's clubs, on radio and television.

Another patient started a stamp collection which developed into a stamp business. Knitting was Ruth's hobby. She, too, started a home business. One year she knitted ninety-six garments.

A hidden talent for drawing was discovered by a myasthenic looking for something to do one afternoon. While thumbing through a magazine she saw a cute picture of two dogs and had the urge to try to draw them. To her surprise she made a creditable reproduction. This spurred her to try other sketching.

You might even try writing that book you have talked about writing or a poem. One patient wrote children's stories which were published. Lois Siemer of Kent, Ohio, wrote *A Patient Speaks:*

> What is joy to me?
> It is so many things
> It is being able to see
> The Beauty that Life brings
>
> It's being able to hold my eyes wide open
> With no double or blurred vision
> To have enough strength to hold a pen
> To have some kind of communication

It's being able to say
The things I want understood
To swallow in an easy way
To chew, if only I could

To be able to lift my head
(without pulling my hair)
From the pillow on my bed
To sit up straight in my chair

To be able to breathe deep
And cough with ease
Not afraid to go to sleep
To get up from my knees

To be able to walk
Without stumbling
To be able to talk
Without stuttering

Why do these mean so much to me?
Because I lost them all
Strength now regained—I'm so happy
To be standing straight and tall

No longer existing from day to day
Not capable of giving
As of today, I am glad to say
I am Now LIVING!

You will need large doses of patience. Patience to wait when the progress is slow. Patience to endure the ignorance of well-meaning friends. There is the one who will slap you on the back and say, "Charley, I know just how you feel. Had the same weakness myself. Now I'll tell you what to do. Get yourself some XYZ pills and take them three times a day. You'll be a new man in a week! Now do as I say. You won't believe it but except for those pills I would be just like you."

Then there is the friend who is always doing things to "get your mind off yourself." She thinks because she is neurotic you are too and therefore imagine all of your weaknesses. There may be the overprotective friend who will smother you with attention.

On the other hand, there will be the faithful, understanding friends who are always ready to give you encouragement and help when needed.

You will need a sense of humor so that you can laugh at your own clumsiness. Laughter is a relaxant. If you become tense and fearful about doing things which require more muscular strength than you think you have, you will have even greater difficulty. For instance, if you are picking up a cup by the handle and this is hard for you, use both hands. If it embarrasses you to do this in

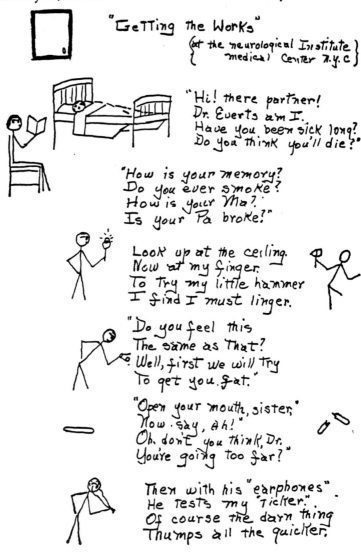

"Getting the Works"
(at the neurological Institute)
(medical Center N.Y.C)

"Hi! there partner!
Dr. Everts am I.
Have you been sick long?
Do you think you'll die?"

"How is your memory?
Do you ever smoke?
How is your Ma?
Is your Pa broke?"

Look up at the ceiling.
Now at my finger.
To try my little hammer
I find I must linger.

"Do you feel this
The same as That?
Well, first we will try
To get you fat."

"Open your mouth, sister."
Now. say, Ah!"
Oh. don't you think, Dr.,
You're going too far?"

Then with his "earphones".
He tests my "Ticker".
Of course the darn thing
Thumps all the quicker.

He thumps my chest.
I say "one, two."
You wonder what's going
To be left of you.

"You'll get a B.C. →(Blood count)
All against your will.
If that don't 'lay you flat'
An L.P. will." ⚡(Lumbar Puncture)

"Maybe a G.I. series→(Gastric Intestinal. Xray series)
And some xrays.
If you're still living
We'll Try one of our G.A.s.→(Gastric Analysis)

Swallow To The Mark.

"How would you like
One of our G.T.T.s→(Glucose Tolerance Test)
We really think
They are the "bees knees".

"Well, I've Tried all my Tricks
No more time need I give
Try as I will
I'm afraid you will live."

So he left me flat.
Closed my chart with a bang.
Says,"I'll see you Friday.
And bring along my Gang."

By Margaret Kirkpatrick

Humor Can Be Found Even in a Hospital

public, if you will jokingly say, "I guess I'd better anchor this cup before it gets away from me," you not only will be at ease but will put the others at ease too.

Days are full of amusing incidents if you look for them. They can even happen in the hospital. One patient wrote about them in the poem, "Getting the Works." Laughter is good medicine and

and will keep you from becoming a sour, grouchy invalid whom people will want to shun. The famous quotation, "Laugh and the world laughs with you. Cry and you cry alone," applies to the myasthenic as well. Remember your illness is the fault of no one. There is no need to make everyone miserable just because you are. A constant complainer or one always talking about his symptoms is a person to be avoided. It is the one who is pleasant, cheerful and uncomplaining who receives respect. "A snapping dog is never petted."

You are apt to have your good days and your bad days. Enjoy the good and tolerate the bad knowing they won't last. One patient kept a variety of projects going which would fit each phase. On bad days when she stayed in bed, she wrote letters, read, listened to special programs or planned a project to do when she was better.

If you expect to feel completely well before you do things, you may never do them. Isn't it too much to expect in any event? Look around you. How many people do you know who never have a pain or ache or are never sick?

Look your best at all times. Just because you feel badly is no excuse to become untidy. Even though you know that your mask-like expression and drooping eyelids eliminate you from being Miss or Mr. America, it is good for your morale to keep well groomed.

One patient reported on the lift she received while hospitalized when she had her hair set in the hospital beauty shop. This encouraged her to put on some makeup. The improvement in her appearance caused people to comment on how much better she looked, which in turn made her feel better.

Keep your emotional health sound. Resolve your problems and get rid of burning resentments even if you must seek professional help. Although you may be physically weak, you can be mentally strong.

Dr. George S. Stevenson, one time National and International Consultant for Mental Health, lists eleven things you can do to preserve your good emotional health:

1. Talk out your trouble with someone in whom you have confidence.

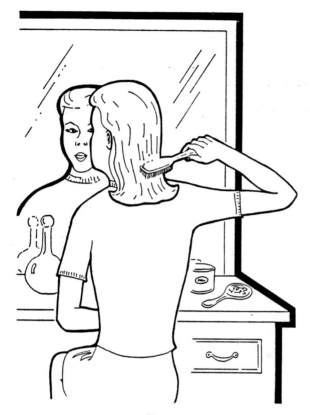

Be Well Groomed

2. When you are upset go off alone until you are composed.
3. When you are angry, work it off.
4. Give in occasionally. You don't always have to be right.
5. Do something for others.
6. Take things one at a time.
7. Shun the "superman" urge.
8. Go easy with your criticism.
9. Give the other fellow a break.

10. Make yourself available by taking the middle between withdrawal and pushing.
11. Schedule your recreation. Everyone needs to play some.

Dr. Stevenson also claims that the philosophy of faith is basic to good emotional health.

Faith in ourselves; faith in others; faith in the ability of each person to improve and grow; faith in the desire and the capacity of human beings to work out their problems cooperatively; faith in the essential decency of mankind, and faith in the great spiritual and moral values. Together they will carry you through stressful situations that might otherwise shatter you.

Your pain is the breaking of the shell
that encloses your understanding.
KAHLIL GIBRAN

4

How To Care For Yourself

†O†O†O†O†O†O†O†O†O†O†O†O†O†O†O†O†O†O†O†O†O†O†O†O†O†O†O†O†O†O

YOU MAY BE fortunate enough to live in or near a large metropolitan area where you can be treated at a medical center or, better still, in a myasthenia gravis clinic. On the other hand, you may be in the country or in a small town and totally dependent on limited medical assistance.

In either case, you are going to have to learn to take care of yourself, to be responsible for your own medicine, to restrict or increase your activity as necessary and to be able to cope with emergencies. Treating myasthenia gravis is something like playing the piano by ear. You have to know certain basic things, but after that, much is governed by feel. Once your illness has been diagnosed and your physician has found the right program for you, he will give you the general rules to follow. Then you are on your own.

No one can actually tell how you should regulate your life. Each has his own mode of living. Certain things which are most essential to one may be of little importance to another. It will,

31

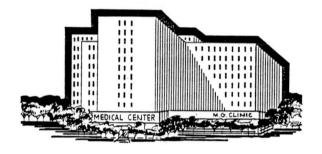

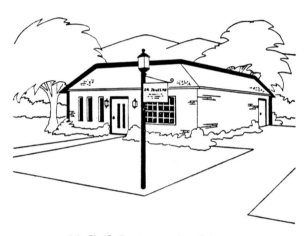

Medical Center or Local Doctor

therefore, be up to you to streamline your living according to your own needs and limitations.

If stairs are difficult, arrange to live on one floor. If you live in a two-floor house, a bed on the first floor may be the thing. This will keep you with the family, the TV and easy access to the out-of-doors. If there is no downstairs bathroom, an inexpensive commode can be bought from a surgical supply store or drugstore. You could even make one by cutting a hole in a wooden box and putting an old-fashioned chamber pot inside it.

For those who spend a lot of time in bed, a backrest and a bed table are good investments. If these cannot be afforded, a heavy cardboard carton cut out to fit over your legs will make a satisfac-

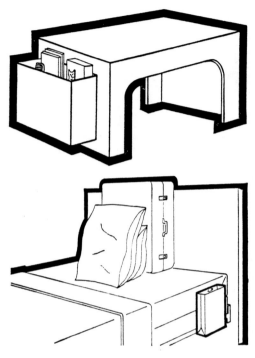

Aids for Comfort

tory substitute. You can have the fun of decorating it with a gay paper. The box should be high enough so that you can rest your arms comfortably and not have to lift them too far to reach your mouth. A smaller box can be stapled to the side of the carton to hold medicine, Kleenex, or whatever you need.

A suitcase can make a passable backrest. Stand it long end up and put a pillow against it. You will find two or three small pillows helpful additions. One for the small of your back and one behind your head will give support for your weak muscles. Pillows under each arm will also relieve the strain if tired.

When lying down, a pillow under the knees is helpful. If light bedcovers bother you, a large pillow placed under the covers at the foot of the bed will keep the covers off your feet. You may prefer to make a leg cradle by cutting two sides from a cardboard carton to fit over your legs. The bedclothes will rest on the box rather than your legs. A foam rubber wedge can be purchased or made to go under the mattress which elevates the head. This is good for those who have weakness in breathing. If one has to be in bed for a long time, one can make stilts from blocks of 4 by 4's. The legs of the bed can fit into these blocks thus elevating the bed for the ease of those caring for you.

You should learn to iron and prepare vegetables sitting down and to write letters, knit, mend, or read while reclining propped up in bed. In other words, sit instead of stand and recline when you don't have to sit.

Do you have difficulty swallowing your pills? If so, pound them in the bottom of a cup, add a little water and drink. Some can be obtained in liquid form. You can also dissolve pills under your tongue. They will work quicker this way.

You will need to learn the response of your medicine so that you have maximum strength when you eat or are physically active. Experience will enable you to know how long it takes you to reach your peak of energy. Then you can gauge the time of good strength before bathing the baby, doing the ironing, mowing the lawn, going to the office or plowing the field. A timer or

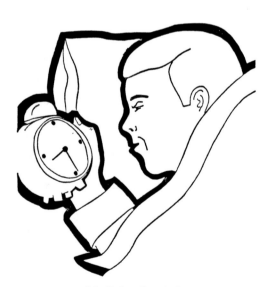

Medicine Reminder

alarm clock is helpful to remind you when to take your medicine. Have you seen the parking meter timers? They are small and fit into a pocket.

It is essential to have your medicine available at all times. You therefore need to keep it within reach. Wear clothes with pockets in the daytime. It is a good idea to count out your pills for the day the first thing in the morning and put them in a small box or vial. It will be easier for you to keep track of the number you have taken. You also can be sure you will not take too many and have a bad reaction.

At night, if you do not have a bedside table, you can keep your night quota of pills under your pillow or in a pajama pocket. If you are prone to respiratory difficulty, it might make you feel easier to have all needed equipment in a paper bag pinned to the side of the bed within easy reach. Those who need to be awakened at night for medication can set an alarm clock. It is a good idea if you are a sound sleeper to have a back-up clock so that the second one will go off if the first one fails to awaken you.

Even though you do not have respiratory weakness, at your doctor's direction and instruction, it may be good to learn to give yourself a hypodermic and to keep a syringe and several ampules on hand in case of an accident or complicating illness, such as pneumonia. If your hands are too weak to give yourself a hypodermic, a member of your family may learn how to give one. This is not as unpleasant as it sounds and the security it will give you will be invaluable.

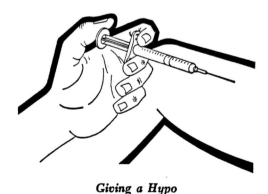

Giving a Hypo

A myasthenic once developed a virus which caused a sudden respiratory difficulty. Her doctor was called but it was two hours before he could be located. While the patient waited for the doctor to come to give her a hypodermic, she came close to panic. This great distress could have been avoided if the patient or her husband had been able to give her the needed medicine hypodermically.

Your doctor or his nurse can teach you how to self-administer your medicine and to sterilize the equipment. Kits, such as diabetics use, can be purchased in the drugstore. They are small enough to fit into a handbag or pocket. It is a good idea to carry one in the pocket of the car as a first-aid measure in case of a bad accident. Of course, your doctor will need to instruct you in the difference between the need for more medicine and an overdose of medicine. Either can produce a severe reaction causing serious weakness.

You will need to protect yourself from viruses. Try to keep yourself built up by eating plenty of good nourishing food, especially the high-protein protective foods. Avoid becoming chilled and exposed to people with colds and illnesses. When influenza is prevalent, stay away from crowds and get extra rest.

Weak spells may follow long exposure to excessive heat or cold. Avoid lying in the sun for a long period or walking far in the cold, especially on a windy day. Too hot baths can be weakening too. Massage and other physical therapy, including a Scotch douche and enemas, should not be used. Strong anger or a "slow burn" over a period of time can be especially weakening so you will need to keep your problems resolved.

Your dentist should be advised of your condition and should call your doctor before giving you any drugs. There are certain ones you should not be given. Myasthenics for instance do not tolerate Novocain® well, or its derivatives. Advise your dentist that you may not be able to hold your mouth open as long as most people. Because your salivary glands may be overactive, the dentist will need to use more swabs to keep the working area dry while he is filling your tooth.

Watch any patent medicine you take. Read the label carefully. A myasthenic should not take anything containing quinine, quinidine, magnesium sulphate, cortisone, thyroid compounds, respiratory depressants, tranquilizers, energizers, morphine or derivatives of curare-like anesthetics.

Be careful about being around when any spraying is done of trees, bushes or plants and do not use spray yourself. Insecticides are anticholinesterase compounds. They inhibit cholinesterase enzymes causing an accumulation of acetylcholine. Avoid using carbon tetrachloride or any cleaning agent that warns about being toxic.

Some patients find smoking weakening, as nicotine can cause toxic reactions. If you smoke, wait until night or a time when you are going to be inactive. Tars may collect in the lungs making breathing more difficult and the treatment of crisis less satisfactory. Alcohol is a depressant and should be left alone. Some myasthenics do not tolerate liquor very well.

If you should have an unexplained slump, look for some unusual symptoms such as fever, sore throat, or pain. Women find they are weakest just prior to or during their menses. At such times, less activity should be planned.

A few patients hesitate to go out socially due to lack of bladder or bowel control. They can feel socially confident by wearing either sanitary napkins with a sanitary shield or incontinent pants with liners. These are available for both men and women in drugstores or surgical supply houses.

Do you have difficulty getting up and down on the commode? Handbars are available. They also come for the shower or tub. A step stool will be a boon for sitting at a sink or workbench. If you look through mailhouse catalogues, you will find a number of gadgets that will make living simpler for you.

If eating is your problem, put a food blender on your Christmas or birthday list. You will be able to concoct all kinds of goodies that will slide down easily. You can also rely on baby food. There is a good variety. It is, however, expensive. The 900-calorie diet drinks might be helpful additions if your eating is limited but should not be relied upon by themselves as a source of food.

You will be able to devise ways of adjusting to your weakness so that you can work and play as strength permits. Although your doctor will advise you and suggest necessary treatment, the suc-

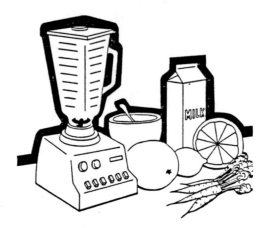

Eating Made Easier

cess of your recovery is dependent upon yourself. You alone will be able to recognize those symptoms which indicate "stop," "rest," or "take a pill." You must be ever on the alert for these warnings and then be wise enough to heed them and take the necessary steps to relieve the symptoms.

You are bound to get discouraged at times and maybe even depressed. Never, however, lose hope. It was Lloyd Douglas who said, "Hope is chuck full of vitamins and far better for you than spinach."

5

How Others Have Managed

✛✚✛

MYASTHENIA GRAVIS is still rare enough that you seldom meet anyone else with the disease unless you are being treated at a clinic or large hospital. For this reason, you do not have a chance to compare notes frequently with another patient. It is often helpful to hear how others are getting along under similar conditions.

No two cases are exactly alike but that does not prevent you from receiving encouragement from the experiences of other myasthenics. Take, for instance, Janice Blake. She is fifty-five, single and developed myasthenia gravis thirty-six years ago. A drooping right eyelid and weakness in her jaw sent her to a medical center. A diagnosis of myasthenia gravis was made.

For a year Janice received ephedrine sulphate, and glycine but showed no improvement. Prostigmin was then given her. Although it did relieve her symptoms, the disease seemed to progress so that more medicine was necessary. Ephedrine was combined with Prostigmin and seemed to give her added strength.

39

As the new drugs came along, Janice tested them all. She seems to do best on Mestinon. On this she is able to work a thirty-hour week in an office. She is not symptom-free but Janice's philosophy is "Do what you want to do, when you want to, and as much as you feel able to. Live as normal a life as possible."

Janice's sister, Mary, also has myasthenia gravis. When Mary was about eighteen, she began developing her weakness. When double vision was added to her drooping eyelids, Janice suspected her sister had myasthenia gravis and took her to a clinic. The diagnosis was confirmed.

As Mary's case was mild, she needed only a minimal amount of Prostigmin. This has enabled Mary to live a normal life. She finds Mestinon more effective. Mary is now married, does all of her own housework, drives a car and takes care of an adopted son.

In speaking about herself, Mary said, "My own case is com-

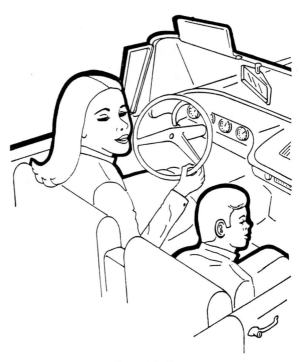

Busy Mother

paratively mild so I just do my best to ignore it. I do what I want to and if the MG makes itself felt, I do only the absolute minimum which means looking after my son. He understands when 'mom is tired.' On those days I prepare simple meals and do very light housework. I rest as much as possible and catch up with reading."

There are two things which Mary has learned to do to make things easier for herself. As she puts it, "I sit down and rest when I'm tired rather than force myself to continue. In the long run my work gets done more quickly and easily that way and I can do more. When people tell me that I look sleepy, I just agree and forget about it. Self-consciousness is about the hardest thing to overcome."

Betty is another patient who developed myasthenia gravis while in her teens. It was in February of 1952, when Betty was sixteen, that she developed a very marked facial weakness, difficulty in swallowing, weakness and difficulty with speech. Her family made the rounds of doctors and hospitals before she got to a myasthenia gravis clinic where the diagnosis was made.

All of the then known medications were tried. Betty tolerated Prostigmin best but had to take massive doses in liquid form and still was very weak. Twice Betty had to be put into a respirator and needed a tube inserted in her throat in order to breathe.

Because Betty had an enlarged thymus, x-ray treatments on the gland were given, but six weeks later it was decided to remove the thymus completely. Six months following the operation Betty had a complete remission and was able to stop all medication. She later secured a position, became active in church and community projects, and married. Betty now has three normal children.

Tom was a myasthenic back in 1935 when he was twenty-five years old. His symptoms developed after an ear infection which was followed by sinusitis. He began having double vision, drooping eyelids and difficulty in talking, smiling and swallowing. It was a year before his condition was correctly diagnosed and relieved by treatment with Prostigmin.

Tom's advice to other myasthenics is, "First, learn to accept it and have someone available, if possible, to give an injection when needed. [His wife gives him his.] Despair and dejection, 'why-did-it-happen-to-me' attitude is bad and usually affects the con-

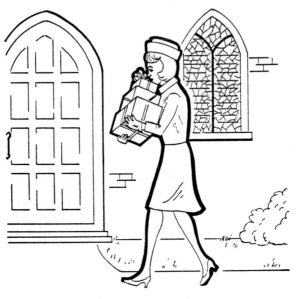

Community Worker

dition adversely. Illness sometimes brings out the best in people. It helped my outlook a lot."

Tom goes on to say the following:

"Of course, I know from my own experience that emotional upsets, virus infections, overexertion and foods not high in protein have an adverse effect on my condition. I have found that alcohol in any form, including in medicines, is very bad for me.

"Moderate smoking is not too bad, but no smoking at all is better for me. Foods high in protein have helped a lot and daily intake of vitamin C, citrus fruit or tomato, have been beneficial. Sometimes breathing becomes very difficult. I have found that keeping as calm as possible and avoiding panic can be the difference between life and death. This breathing difficulty generally occurred during or after a virus attack."

Charles, another myasthenic, works as a watchman, walking five miles a day, five days a week. One day he walks thirteen miles. He couldn't do that back in 1938 for he had weakness in walking, talking, breathing and eating. At the time he was diagnosed, all medications were tried but he did best on Prostigmin.

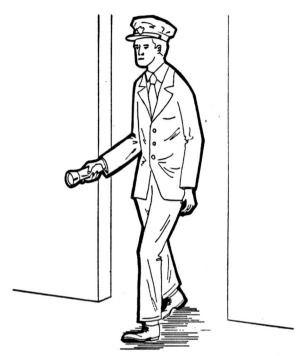

The Night Watchman

He had a seven-year remission. Charles learned that by setting his mind to doing something and trying to take it in easy stages and working along slowly, he could do it. Match cover collecting is his hobby.

A patient of sixty first experienced pain in the back of her head, weakness in her arms and legs and drooping eyelids. She required large amounts of Mestinon daily plus potassium chloride. Her advice is "keep yourself busy with a part-time job, if possible. Cultivate a hobby which does not require too much energy but with enough interest to keep your mind occupied." Knitting is this patient's hobby.

If you think you have had a runaround, you should meet Sally. She had myasthenia gravis for thirteen years before it was diagnosed. It all began during the early years of her marriage. Although she was not very active, she was exhausted all the time.

Flu, followed by pneumonia, nearly finished her. She became pregnant and grew worse again. Because of irritability, nervousness and depression, she was given stilbestrol. When this did not help, she was sent to a psychiatrist who sent her back to the gynecologist.

Rheumatoid arthritis put her in a cast for three months, then a Taylor brace for three years. The prolonged use of stilbestrol caused a condition which required a curettage. This was followed by the removal of an ovarian cyst and a partial hysterectomy. The weakness was eventually diagnosed as myasthenia gravis and treated with Prostigmin. Sally had a hard time getting the dosage regulated. Mestinon was tried. This proved better for her. It enables her to do her own housework, teach knitting and to go out occasionally. She warns, "Don't push yourself too far. Don't expect anyone to understand your disease or your struggles except your doctor. Learn to get along all day by yourself if you have to. Try to get really interested in something that will keep you fascinated and won't take much energy. It makes days pass much more quickly."

It would do you good to see Virginia energetically walking down the street. She is a young-looking middle-aged woman who developed myasthenia gravis about twenty years ago. Her symptoms included dizziness, inability to focus her eyes properly, drooping eyelids, weakness of limbs, extreme fatigue, difficulty with speech, swallowing, a "tightness in the head" causing a "couldn't think" feeling. The Prostigmin test confirmed the diagnosis. She took Prostigmin without much benefit. Large doses made her worse. She spent most of her time lying in bed or sitting in a chair.

Virginia became interested in nutrition. Just prior to her illness, she had dieted rather rigidly to lose weight and began to wonder if this had anything to do with her illness. After reading all of the books on nutrition available in the library, Virginia decided to try raising the standard of her own diet. She went on a high-protein, high-vitamin diet and added high-potency vitamin supplements. Now Virginia needs no Prostigmin or other anticholinergic medicine and lives a very full life.

Bernice, fifty, and her twenty-eight-year-old son have myasthenia gravis. Bernice lost her voice completely for six months. For a while her eyelids drooped so badly they finally closed completely. Mestinon time-span tablets proved best for her. Her son's case was diagnosed before his illness developed beyond the severe fatigue stage. He needs only a few Mestinon daily.

Elsie tells her story this way. "I have had M.G. for about sixteen years. My first symptoms were difficulty in talking and swallowing. I went to a throat specialist. She suggested I have my tonsils removed. After I had my tonsils taken out and my speech and swallowing had not improved, I went to my family doctor who immediately diagnosed my illness as M.G. He put me on Prostigmin."

Following a bout with a virus, Elsie developed double pneumonia and required ten days of respiratory assistance. Elsie has taken a variety of the drugs but likes Mytelase best. She works in a busy office, leads an active social life and travels alone all around the country.

These are but a few of thousands of cases who have made the uphill climb. There are those who cannot be as active as some of these people but, as their case stories show, it took some a long time to get to their active state. Although the symptoms and experiences of these case stories differ, the people all had a good attitude. They learned to live with their illness in a way to bring satisfactions and a feeling of fulfillment. Maybe it is because their hearts are open. Jane Austin said, "Everybody's heart is open, you know, when they have recently escaped from severe pain, or are recovering the blessing of health."

6

Childhood Myasthenia Gravis

As early as 1877 it was recognized that children could have myasthenia gravis. There are an ever-increasing number of cases being seen. Up to 1900 eight cases were reported. Now, in just one large clinic, 11 percent of all patients seen are children or infants.

There are two kinds of childhood myasthenia gravis: neonatal and congenital. Neonatal myasthenia gravis occurs when the mother is a myasthenic. This is detected at birth or within a few days. It lasts only a few weeks and usually does not reoccur.

About 20 percent of myasthenic mothers have myasthenic infants which may have difficulty in sucking, a weak cry, difficulty in breathing, weakness in moving extremities and an expressionless face.

Neostigmine (Prostigmin) or pyridostigmine is given. Of course, smaller doses are given to infants. Great care must be taken to avoid overdosage which will cause such side reactions as diarrhea, vomiting, rapid heartbeat, excessive salivary secretions and in severe reactions, heart arrest.

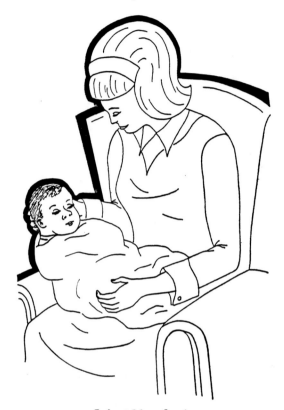

Infant Myasthenic

Because the mother's anticholinesterase medication can be transferred through her breast milk, the baby cannot be breast fed. It must be put on a formula and "preemie nipples" used.

In neonatal myasthenia gravis it is thought there is a passage of a "myasthenia factor" of antibody nature across the placenta. Intensive studies are being carried out to isolate this factor. Often the mother has another child who also has neonatal myasthenia gravis.

Congenital myasthenia gravis or juvenile myasthenia gravis, as it is sometimes called, occurs in infants and children up to fourteen years of age. Their mothers are non-myasthenic. Unlike neonatal myasthenia, it persists and is apt to be permanent. Al-

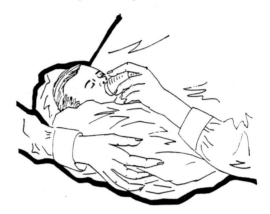

Feeding the Infant with Preemie Bottle

though the disease is not inherited, more than one child in a family may have it.

Most of the children have generalized weakness. They tire easily and cannot keep up in sports. Some children, however, have only eye symptoms. Generally the symptoms are bilateral in that they affect both eyes, both hands, or both legs.

As in neonatal myasthenia, the same medicines are used in the smaller doses and care must be taken not to overdose. Some parents give more medicine in an effort to increase activity. This could cause a respiratory crisis. In this case the anticholinesterase drug is withdrawn for seventy-two hours and the respiration supported if necessary. Fewer children than adults have crises. Children respond well to treatment. Most have to be treated continuously. A few have had complete freedom of symptoms.

Myasthenia gravis in infants is quite rare and fortunately is usually mild. However, caring for an infant with myasthenia gravis is a twenty-four–hour job according to a mother of twins who have myasthenia gravis. The mother, father and grandparents divide the twenty-four hours into shifts so that one is available to care for the babies at all times. Each has developed an awareness of a special sound or grunt which indicates trouble. They try to anticipate the baby's need to avoid its crying. Crying will increase a breathing hazard and may bring on a crisis.

As a baby needs to be observed at all times, it is good to replace the nursery door with one that is half glass. A low night light will enable one to observe at night without opening the door. An intercom in the nursery will help to amplify his breathing and you will be able to hear a weak cry or a choking sound caused by an accumulation of saliva in the throat which may need to be aspirated.

It is helpful to keep the head higher. With a portable crib, the legs of the headboard can be extended. If this kind is not available, one can put a pillow under the mattress at the head or use

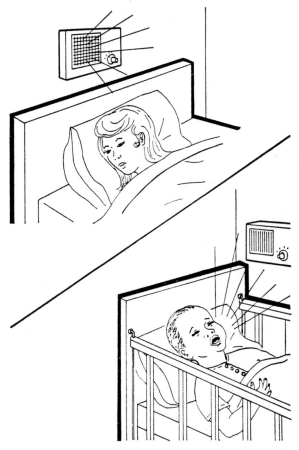

For Cries in the Night

a foam rubber wedge. The baby should never be laid flat or on its stomach if it has any breathing weakness. If one lives in a hot, humid climate an air conditioner in the nursery will make life more comfortable and breathing easier.

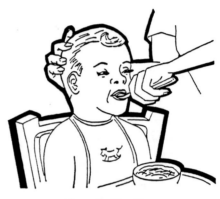

Care in Feeding

Extra time is needed in feeding a myasthenic infant or child. Allow for rest periods and watch to be sure he is able to swallow all that is being given. If not, stop and allow him to rest before continuing.

It is wise to know how to give medication by hypodermic and keep an ample supply of ampules on hand as well as two tanks of oxygen in case of a crisis. Know the difference between the crisis of an overdose of medication and the need for more medicine.

Learn what helps the baby to relax quickly—rocking, warm towels on legs, patting or singing. Each baby has its own responses. It is important to be able to relax him quickly if he gets overexcited, has a choking spell or difficulty in breathing.

Avoid taking the baby into crowds and ask people not to visit if they have colds or do not feel well. The baby must be guarded against infections of all kinds. See that his head and back are supported when sitting. Avoid rough play, prolonged play or any activity that is tiring. However, a baby needs to be played with, sung to, read to and loved like any infant, only for shorter periods.

A myasthenic child has other problems. One little girl failed reading because her teacher did not know the girl had myasthenia gravis and her double vision made reading difficult for her. The teacher, playmates and those with whom the child is in frequent contact should be told of the illness and any limitations. The child may need to be excused from strenuous exercise in school and active sports. He should be given ample opportunity to excel, however, in areas in which he can achieve without overfatigue.

One must avoid overprotectiveness and develop self-confidence in the child. He needs to feel secure in the family and in his relationship with others. Spoiling will bring on temper tantrums which are very weakening. Help the child live as normal a life as possible. Childhood is such a happy time; keep it so for the myasthenic infant and child.

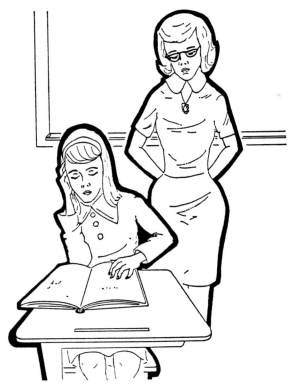

Reading Problems

How beautiful is youth! How bright
its gleams
With illusions, aspirations, dreams!
Book of beginning, story without end,
Each maid a heroine, and each man
a friend!

H. W. Longfellow

7

Tips For Teenagers

+○

IT IS HARD ENOUGH to get through the troublesome teen years
when one is well, but to have myasthenia gravis and be a teenager is a real challenge. First, you will need to know all you can
about your illness. If you concentrate on getting your medication
regulated so that activity can be more or less continuous without
big slumps, you have it made and will be able to enjoy many of
the teen frolics.

As far as sports are concerned, it would be wise for you to be
content to be a good spectator rather than an active participant.
Each sport needs a good cheering squad. You can be the best
booster. You may be able to play some active games provided you
aren't in competition and can stop when you start to tire. The
same thing is true of swimming. Be careful, though, about going
into deep water. Your legs and arms might suddenly weaken and
you would be in serious trouble getting to the shore or out of the
pool. Never swim alone.

Everyone has his particular interest and talent. You should be
able to develop yours provided you do not go to extremes. No
matter how great you are at your special interest, someone else
is always going to be better than you are so there is no need to
push too hard just to be at the top. Cool the big drive bit.

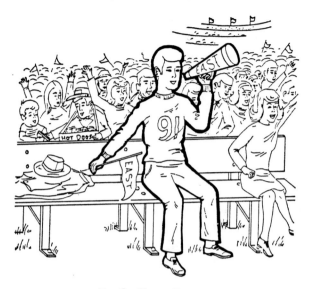

Be the Team Booster

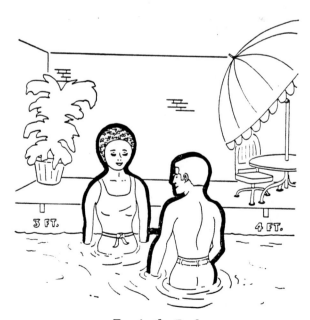

Fun in the Pool

It is natural for young adults to want to be on the go all the time and to be part of a noisy crowd. No one wants to be called "chicken." Young people can be cruel to each other. Not because they mean to be but because they do not understand. To save yourself embarrassment and crushed feelings, be frank with your friends and let them know you have an unusual illness and may have to drop out of activity suddenly. Be sure, however, you do not use myasthenia gravis as an excuse to duck out of things you do not want to do.

Each person has a certain amount of energy to spend in a day. How you spend it is largely your choice. Because you may be a little short on energy sometimes, it is wise to learn to budget your time as one does money. Do the must things first. Things less important may be held over until tomorrow.

Keeping up with school is a must. You will need to finish high school in order to go on to either college or a vocational school. Because you have a physical limitation, vocational rehabilitation will help you to get additional education. Ask your school counselor or employment security counselor for more information.

You will need to look ahead to the time when you will be able to get a job and become self-supporting. Think in terms of a career which uses more brain than brawn. There is no need to wallow in self-pity and expect to be waited on the rest of your life. Get with it. Look ahead to a good career.

One of the big deals all young adults have to face is to smoke or not to smoke; to drink or not to drink. Both are out for you. The answer is simple. No, No, No! The nicotine in cigarettes is a toxic substance which interferes with the acetylcholine-cholinesterase balance and will cause you to weaken and will make your heart beat faster. The alcohol in liquor, even beer, acts as a depressant and will weaken your muscular control faster than the average person's. If your friends call you a square if you don't drink or smoke, keep your cool. They aren't even worthy of being called friends. True friends will understand and will not urge or tease you. Remember too, experimentation with pot, goof balls, LSD or any drugs not ordered by your doctor is apt to take you on a trip with no return. Forget it!

Dating is an important part of your teen years. Love need not pass you by. You still can be a good date but play the love game cool. You can look ahead to marriage but don't rush it. Enjoy your teen years as a time to have many dating partners. A time to find out the kind of partner which is best suited to you.

For you, girls, you will need to find a boy who is especially considerate. One who will be willing to wait on you should the occasion arise. A boy who will not push you beyond your endurance and is flexible enough to give up a date should you not feel up to going dancing.

You young man will need to look for the kind of partner who will make a sweet, understanding wife. One who will not urge you to take her places when you are too tired. A girl who can assume responsibility and is a hard worker, capable of earning a living for both if necessary. She should be able to keep her head in an emergency and find satisfaction in blending activity with quiet periods. She should like to stay home evenings instead of always wanting to be going somewhere.

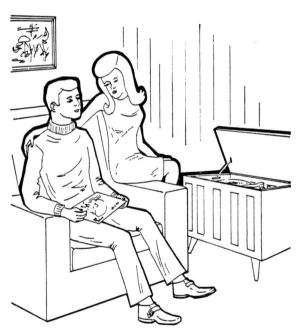

Choosing the Right Partner

It is going to take you longer to find your just right mate. So what if you have to watch your friends marry and you feel left out. You won't have the regrets they may experience. Teen marriages may seem romantic but most end in divorce.

Suppose you are one of the less fortunate ones who has a difficult time adjusting to your medicine and your weakness prevents you from going to school or keeping up with the gang. You can keep up with your schoolwork at home by having friends bring you assignments and by talking to your teachers by phone. There are always those willing to tutor especially if you are willing to show some effort.

Learn to budget your time. Instead of crowding yourself, allow plenty of time to do each task so you will not be under pressure and have to hurry. Most teenagers act as though they were jet propelled. You are going to need to balance your daily routine by sandwiching periods of quiet and relaxation between your periods of activity. There is nothing drastic about this and it is certainly better than goofing off and doing nothing.

Myasthenia gravis may slow you down a bit but it need not destroy your sense of humor, your spirit of challenge, your friendliness, good sportsmanship or ambition. It will not sap your talents, need not sour your disposition or send you into a tailspin of despair. You cannot run away from it, shrug it off or wish it away. Accept it and adjust to living with it. Play it smart and follow the doctor's orders as though he were a sergeant in the army. Then get out and face the world as you are even if you see it double. Life can still be fun, full of the unexpected, exciting and rewarding. You, though, have a major role in making it so.

Those who have the largest hearts
have the soundest understandings:
and he is the truest philosopher who
can forget himself.

WILLIAM HAZLITT

8

For Friends, Relatives and Parents

+O+O+O+O+O+O+O+O+O+O+O+O+O+O+O+O+O+O+O+O+O+O+O+O+O+O+O+O+O

A FRIEND, relative or parent can be the key figure in keeping up the morale of a person suffering from a long, serious illness. To be ill in any way is difficult. To have a strange, baffling disease such as myasthenia gravis is especially hard. It is more difficult to battle the unknown.

Everyone has experienced the miseries of the flu or a sore throat. Many have had some kind of operation. Mention arthritis or polio and you find a kindred feeling of understanding. Mention myasthenia gravis and people look at you in bewilderment and say, "Myasthenia gravis? What in the world is that?" It makes the patient feel like some kind of freak.

It is even harder for the patient to describe his symptoms. How can one explain that the fatigue in myasthenia gravis is different from the feeling that comes from a day of housecleaning or playing 18 holes of golf on a hot day? How can one describe the kind of fatigue that seems to pierce the very marrow of the bone and make any movement seem impossible?

Who can imagine the despair that goes with being hungry,

wanting to eat, yet finding each taunting bite a monumental mouthful to chew and swallow. With each swallow there is danger of choking. Have you ever choked on a fish bone or gotten something stuck in your throat? Do you remember suddenly being unable to breathe and the struggle that ensued? This may happen to you once in a lifetime but the experience is etched in your mind. A myasthenic who has great difficulty in swallowing may have had several such experiences and have to limit himself to eating baby food in order to prevent serious choking attacks.

Have you ever wanted desperately to do something, to go somewhere, but were so weak you couldn't even fasten a pin? This could be the way a myasthenic feels. Unless you have the disease yourself, you have never gone through the misery and anxieties connected with it.

It is very important that you refrain from such phrases as "I know how you feel." "You could make yourself do it if you wanted to." "Snap out of it!" "Get your mind off of yourself and you'll feel better." These are cruel remarks and all untrue. A myasthenic, first of all, needs to feel your acceptance of him as he is. He needs your companionship, the warmth of your understanding almost as much as he needs his medicine. He needs to be treated, as much as possible, like a well person and not constantly reminded of his limitations.

Be tactful about shielding in an obvious way and causing him to feel conspicuous. Be alert to signs of weakening if you are out together and make an excuse that you are tired and would like to stop a while.

Allow plenty of time for things you are going to do together so you do not have to rush. Avoid pushing a myasthenic beyond his endurance; you cannot depend upon your own fatigue as a barometer of his. Just do not keep at one thing too long. See that there are places to sit down when you are at a gathering or out walking.

Myasthenics whose facial muscles are affected are aware that their unusual facial expression, drooping lids and difficulty in smiling give them an unpleasant appearance. They tend to be sensitive about it. You can help a girl or woman feel more attractive by giving her gifts of pretty clothes, cosmetics, perfume and,

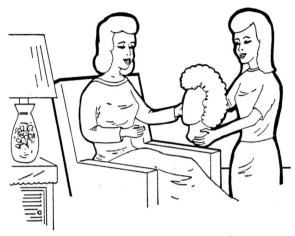

A Wig Is a Thoughtful Gift

for some, a pretty wig will do wonders. The effort of combing hair and keeping it attractively styled is a very great strain on weak arm and hand muscles.

In choosing clothes as gifts, avoid ones with small buttons to be fastened and those that slip over the head. Cardigan sweaters are better than pullovers. Loosely fitted clothes go on easier than tight fitting ones. Look for front fastenings rather than back. For men, pre-tied ties are a boon.

Become as well informed as possible but understand that each patient is an individual whose symptoms may be different from another. With early diagnosis, most patients live fairly normal lives. There are some, however, who have difficulty adjusting to medicine and may have trouble judging the amount needed. Taking too much can be as bad as taking too little. You need to recognize the symptoms of each kind of reaction and know what to do about it.

You can do a lot to keep the patient optimistic, encouraged and confident. He naturally is going to have periods of discouragement. See that he doesn't become a recluse. If he doesn't go out much, bring activity to him. Arrange for surprises. Keep him informed about what is going on so he won't feel left out of everything.

When the myasthenic is able to get out, see that he is included in invitations to various events he enjoys. Many public places where much walking is required now have wheelchairs available. If, for instance, your myasthenic is a football fan, a call ahead to the stadium would verify if a wheelchair is available. Permission can generally be obtained for driving the car to an entrance close to your seats. Choose seats that do not require a lot of steep climbing.

When traveling by plane or train you can avoid the long fatiguing walk to and from the plane or train by notifying the passenger agent of the need of a wheelchair. The patient can safely travel alone.

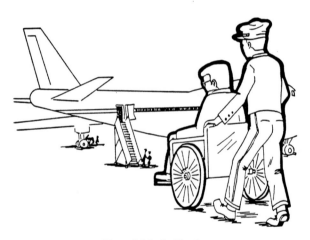

Travel Made Easier

When the myasthenic travels by car, a headrest or neck pillow will make his trip more comfortable. Plan trips for morning rather than late afternoon. In a two-door car, it is easier for him to sit in the front seat. On a long trip, frequent stops, rests and snacks will make the trip less tiring.

For the patient who drives, power steering and power brakes are a big help. If a person is not troubled by double vision and is not in a seriously weakened condition, he should have no problem about driving.

Remember that simple little things like opening heavy doors, jar lids, carrying trays in a restaurant, stooping, pulling on a girdle, gloves or even fastening a pin may be extremely difficult for some myasthenics. Be patient if it takes him longer. If you can do it without offense, you might be considerate and help him.

If a myasthenic has speech difficulty and you find it hard understanding him, listen very intently and be as close as you can to catch every word. Try to avoid having him repeat everything. It is not only exhausting for him but very frustrating as well.

A fretting, anxious person around a myasthenic can be irritating and weakening. He has enough anxieties of his own without absorbing yours. What he needs from you is calmness, strength, patience, encouragement and a good sense of humor. Many people have little patience with those who are ill. This hostile attitude is generally due to a lack of knowledge of the problem. It is a reaction to the illness rather than to the patient.

A myasthenic has bad days as well as good ones. There may be days when he is a grouch and nothing seems to please him. Try though, without spoiling him, to avoid serious emotional conflicts with him. They can be weakening. The myasthenic needs to recognize that his illness is hard on his family and friends too and try to be considerate and cooperative.

It must be remembered that while the myasthenic may be ill, weak and even have difficulty in communicating, he has the same intelligence he had prior to his illness. He very much resents being treated like a moron, being dominated and having people constantly telling him what he can and cannot do. He needs to keep his mind stimulated, his interests developed and be allowed to be as independent as possible.

You will need to resist making a chronic invalid out of him. You understand that recovery may be slow. It will be a long, hard pull for all. You are a vital part of a lifesaving team. Like any team work, it takes cooperation, coordination, determination, faith and hope to get the best results.

To suffer and endure is a lot of hu-
manity.

Pope Leo XIII

No pain, no palm: No thorns, no
throne:
No gall, no glory: No cross, no crown.

William Penn

9

What To Do In An Emergency

+O+O+O+O+O+O+O+O+O+O+O+O+O+O+O+O+O+O+O+O+O+O+O+O+O+O+O+O+O+O+O

D UE TO early diagnosis and management, few myasthenics now
go through the critical aspects of the disease. However, like
everyone else, a myasthenic can develop other illnesses which can
complicate his condition. A bad bout with a virus, pneumonia or
the need for extensive surgery could cause special problems.

To know what to do in an emergency is more than half of the
battle, for one needs to keep calm, work quickly and have all
needed equipment conveniently at hand. To be prepared is something like fire prevention exercises in schools. Children are taught
what to do in case of fire and have repeated drills. Seldom is their
knowledge put to use. The few times it is used, lives are saved.

It is mandatory for family members to learn from their physician what to do in the case of emergencies. Suppose a myasthenic
has difficulty swallowing and suddenly chokes on a bit of food,
what would you do? Just hitting him on the back is not enough.
In a myasthenic, the salivary glands become overactive and the
saliva accumulates, blocking the airway.

First, the patient should not panic. He or someone else should try to put their fingers down his throat and pull out whatever is lodged there. Generally it can be reached. While this is being done a member of the family can be pumping air into his lungs by raising his arms up and down, in rapid succession. It will take a concerted effort of all present to help if the food cannot be dislodged. One should call a rescue squad or ambulance and then the doctor. While waiting, use an aspirator.

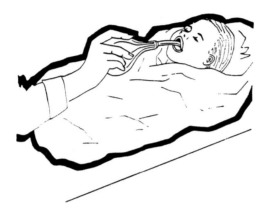

Using an Aspirator

An aspirator is a handy gadget to keep on hand for any patient who has trouble chewing. You can get them at the drugstore for about two dollars. An aspirator is a rubber-ball-like object with a long, curved tube extended from it. One inserts this gently into the throat and squeezes the bulb in and out to take up the saliva.

If you do not have a rescue squad or ambulance or you are unable to reach your doctor for instructions and there is a hospital within a few miles, carry the patient to the car. Under no circumstances let him walk. Prop him up with pillows and open all of the windows. Let the emergency room of the hospital know you are coming. Also, call the police or sheriff. They will meet you and clear the road for you. Be calm and quiet but move quickly.

Even though your myasthenic may never need emergency treatment it is a good idea for you to give the police, sheriff and the rescue squad written instructions from your doctor.

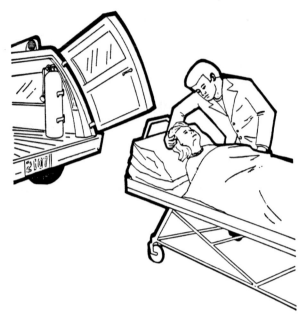

Emergency Help

If you live a distance from a hospital, there are home respirators that can be used for such emergencies. There is a hand-operated one that sells for a moderate price and is available from a surgical supply house. More elaborate ones are also available on a loan basis should your myasthenic develop complications such as pneumonia and has difficulty breathing.

It is good for a member of the family to know how to give mouth-to-mouth resuscitation. This can help a myasthenic experiencing cardiac arrest until mechanical assistance is available. If a patient should have a respiratory crises which you recognize is due to lack of medication but you are unable to give a hypo, have the patient put an anticholinesterase pill under his tongue. You may have to do it for him. There will be enough saliva to dissolve the pill. Gently stroke the throat. This will help him to swallow. Keep your fingers on his pulse and watch the patient's color. If he begins to look blue around the mouth, start mouth-to-mouth resuscitation.

Some patients develop a sense of security by learning how to give themselves a hypo. Their doctors teach them how to do this. There are traveling diabetic kits that can be carried in the purse or pocket. One patient who has traveled extensively always takes her hypodermic kit with her, confident that she will be able to handle any unforeseen emergency which might arise due to an accident or illness while in a strange place. An emergency kit and a few anticholinesterase pills should be carried in the pocket of

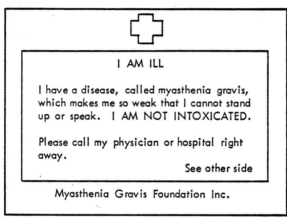

FRONT

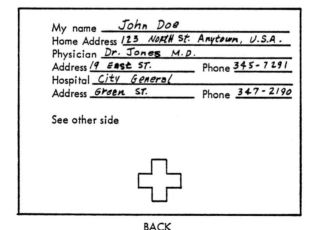

BACK

Myasthenia Gravis Emergency Card

the car with instructions for use. It is a good idea for the patient to carry emergency care instructions in his purse or wallet. Of course, all myasthenics should wear a medical alert tag of some kind to call attention to the fact that they have myasthenia gravis. In addition, the patient should carry a letter from his physician with instructions for care. The Myasthenia Gravis Foundation, Inc., will send special identification cards for myasthenics upon request.

Even patients who are in remission should carry emergency instructions. One such patient needed surgery, which was to be performed by a surgeon living some distance from the patient's regular physician. The surgeon had such difficulty believing that the patient was a myasthenic and needed special precautions taken that the patient could not take a chance on his doing the operation. She traveled a long distance to be under the supervision of the doctor who knew her condition. A well-meaning but uninformed doctor can do a patient a great deal of harm. Too few have had experience with the disease and welcome instructions from the attending physician.

Choking episodes can be prevented or minimized if a patient avoids fish with bones in it, nuts and foods difficult to chew or that have a stringy residue like stringy meat and celery. Also, while the myasthenic is eating, consideration should be given about teasing, making the patient talk a lot or making him laugh.

The patient who needs help may be in such a weakened condition that he has difficulty making himself heard. The person caring for him should be alert for strange sounds, weak calls, a tap on the table top. Keeping a hand bell within reach of the patient is helpful.

If a myasthenic weakens while in the sun, carry him to the shade, put cold compresses on his head and loosen his clothes. If he is able to swallow, give him sips of a cool drink. If he weakens while in the cold, carry him to a warm room and give a hot drink.

Fear of dying is something any seriously ill person has, especially of dying unnecessarily. If he is confident that those around him know how to cope with an emergency, he is not apt to panic. The calmness, love and understanding of those with him can do much to relieve his fear.

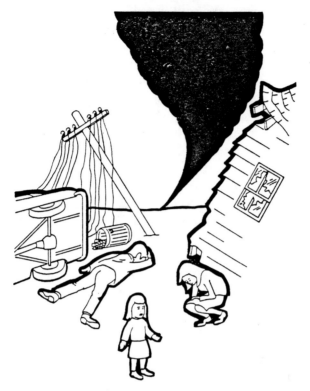

Preparedness Can Prevent Disaster

Everyone and everything must die sometime. In this we are all equal. No one escapes. We live constantly with death. A tornado suddenly sweeps down and kills. Fire, floods, lightning and disease sometimes bring death without warning. Life is but a temporary phase in the cycle of being, yet each life contributes to the total universe. Each lives on into eternity through his acts. In the Old Testament, Chapter 3 of Ecclesiastes beautifully expresses this idea: To everything there is a season, and a time for every purpose under the heavens; a time to be born and a time to die. John Ruskin wrote, "Every noble life leaves the fiber of it interwoven forever in the work of the world."

Whole civilizations have been buried. Archeologists are digging them out. Although centuries ago, the people of those times have had a direct bearing on our lives today. The same is true of us in future generations. Each myasthenic also plays an important role in the advancement of medical science. No myasthenic will ever die in vain.

Some myasthenics have another kind of fear, the fear of living with a baffling disease, the fear of losing friends as a result. A few patients have been divorced by their mates as a result of their illness. Some fear being a burden to their families, and worry about how their illness is going to be financed. To them death is the only release. They either lose the will to live or they deliberately induce death in one way or another. Periods of deep depression or threats of wanting to die should be viewed with concern and extra love and attention given. It may be necessary to seek psychiatric help.

Epicurus once said a long time ago, "It is not so much our friend's help that helps us as the confidence of their help." This confidence can dispel many of the myasthenic's fears. It can help a critical situation become just an unusually active period instead of a dire emergency. So much depends upon the confidence of that help.

It is part of the cure to wish to be
cured.

SENECA: Phaedra c. 60

10

Where To Go For Help

†O†O†O†O†O†O†O†O†O†O†O†O†O†O†O†O†O†O†O†O†O†O†O†O†O†O†O†O†O†O

THIRTY-FIVE years ago few doctors had heard of myasthenia
gravis. It was a disease mentioned in a medical book but
seldom seen. The door of encouragement in the United States for
increased research was opened with the publication of the paper,
*The Oral Use of Prostigmin in the Treatment of Myasthenia
Gravis* by Dr. William Everts.

The first myasthenia gravis clinic was opened by Dr. Viets in
1935 at the Massachusetts General Hospital in Boston. Today
there are twenty-one clinics devoted entirely to myasthenia gravis
and new ones are opening all the time.

The increased interest in the disease, the number of clinics and
the amount of research being done can be attributed largely to
the work of the Myasthenia Gravis Foundation, Inc. It started in
1952 as a dream of a mother determined to get help for her
daughter.

The mother, Jane Ellsworth, realized that only through research and the dissemination of information could the ultimate
cure be found for this baffling disease. She knew some kind of an
organization was necessary to collect and distribute the information. Money, too, was important to be used for research.

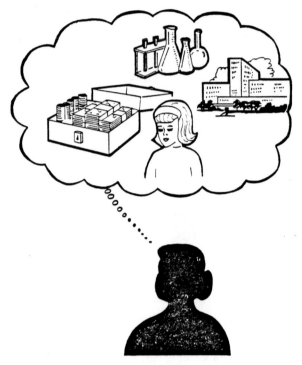

One Woman's Dream

Beginning in her husband's office and with a few faithful friends, Mrs. Ellsworth started a one woman campaign which resulted in the formation of the Myasthenia Gravis Foundation, Inc. It is located in the Academy of Medicine Building, 2 East 103rd Street, New York, New York.

The foundation has six goals:

1. To foster, coordinate and support research into the cause, prevention, alleviation and cure of myasthenia gravis.
2. To give voluntary aid and assistance in every lawful and honorable manner to the sufferers of this disease.
3. To disseminate among the members of the medical profession, information concerning the results of research into myasthenia gravis, as well as information concerning advances in therapeutic procedures.
4. To disburse research funds to institutions and individuals

at any time and from time to time, for the purpose of carrying out their objectives and for the prevention, diagnosis, treatment, alleviation or cure of myasthenia gravis and related diseases.

5. To publicize in every dignified, factual and honorable way the characteristics of myasthenia gravis and information concerning research and therapy.

6. To cooperate with other corporations engaged in similar activities, with a view toward carrying out the objectives herein described above.

There are local chapters of the Myasthenia Gravis Foundation, Inc., in most states of the United States. Each chapter works hard to raise money for research, provide education and services for the myasthenic. Because of the dependency of many patients on a large number of pills a day, the cost of purchasing them is beyond their means. Many chapters have pill banks where the needed medicine can be bought at a low cost.

Another large service of the local chapter is providing the myasthenic with a feeling he is not alone, struggling with a baffling disease. Through chapter meetings, the myasthenic has a chance to learn how other myasthenics manage the disease. He finds inspiration and hope.

If you do not live near a treatment center or a myasthenia gravis chapter, your doctor can receive information concerning the most advanced methods of treatment by writing to the foundation headquarters. The foundation publishes a newsletter with latest research findings and *A Handbook for Patients*. These are available on request. You might like to join a chapter even though it is not near you and buy your medicine at low prices. You can obtain the address of the chapter nearest you by writing to the foundation office.

It is a real inspiration and incentive for you to learn how other patients meet their weaknesses. Only someone else who has been through similar experiences can share your feelings. Some chapters have lists of patients who want to correspond with other patients.

Do not hesitate to ask questions. The national foundation headquarters or the chapter office nearest you will be glad to answer them. Tennyson once said, "Faith, I think, begins only when we start to ask questions. Faith is not what you know. What you know is fact. Faith is what you go on when you don't know."

This is what you have to go on from here. Faith in the future of myasthenia gravis. Faith in the doctors and scientists all over the world who are working zealously to find a cure; who keep searching for the answers. Faith in your physician and, most of all, faith in yourself. With this faith, myasthenia gravis will be conquered!

Bibliography

Adams, M., Power, M. H., and Boothby Walter, M.: Chemical studies of myasthenia gravis. *Ann Intern Med, 9*:823, 1936.

Aeschlimann, John A., and Reinert, Marc: The pharmacological action of some analogues of physostigmine. *J Pharmacol, 43*:413–444, 1931.

Alpert, L. I., Papatestas, A., Kark, A., Osserman, R. S., and Osserman, K.: A histologic reappraisal of the thymus in myasthenia gravis. A correlative study of thymic pathology and response to thymectomy. *Arch Pathol, 91*:55–61, 1971.

Arnett, C. J., and Ritchie, J. M.: The ionic requirements for the action of acetylcholine on mammalian non-myelinated fibres. *J Physiol, 165*: 141–159, 1963.

Bergh, Nils P.: Biologic assays in myasthenia gravis for any agents causing neuromuscular block. *Scand J Clin Lab Invest 5*:5–47, 1953.

Beutner, E. H.: Myasthenia gravis: Primary auto-immunity still unclear. *Med Tribune,* June 13–14, 1964.

Billig, Jr., Harvey E., and Morehouse, L. E.: Performance and metabolic alteration during betaine glycocyamine feeding in myasthenia gravis. *Arch Phys Med, 36*:233, 1965.

Blalock, A., Mason, M. F., Morgan, H. J., and Riven, S. S.: Myasthenia gravis and tumors of the thymic region. *Ann Surg, 110*:544, 1939.

Blaugrund, S. M.: Studies in myasthenia gravis. The role of tracheotomy and controlled ventilation. *Ann Otol, 73*:618–631, 1964.

Booker, H. E.; Chun, Raymond, W. M., and Sanguino, Miguel: Myasthenia

73

gravis syndrome associated with trimethadione. *JAMA, 212*:2262–2263, 1970.

Boothby, W. M.: Myasthenia gravis. Effect of treatment with glycine and ephedrine. (5th report) *Proc Staff Meet Mayo Clinic, 9*:593–597, 1934.

Cambier, J.: Myasthenia. II Physiopathology, diagnosis and treatment. *Presse Med (Paris), 65*:737–740, 1957.

Chafetz, Morris E.: Psychological disturbances in myasthenia gravis. *Ann NY Acad Sci, 135*:424–427, 1966.

Cherington, M. Neonatal myasthenia gravis. *Lancet, 1*:570, 1969.

Cumming, J. N.: The role of potassium in myasthenia gravis. *J Neurol Neurosurg Psychiat, 3*:115, 1940.

Dawson, J. R. B.: Myasthenia gravis in a cat. *Vet Rec, 86*:562–563, 1970.

Denny-Brown, D.: Neurological conditions resulting from prolonged severe dietary restrictions. *Medicine, 26*:41–113, 1947.

Deutsch, Ronald W.: The mysterious disease of weakness. *Ladies Home Journal reprint*, Curtis Publishing Co., 1956.

Edgeworth, Harriet: A report of progress in the use of ephedrine in a case of myasthenia gravis. *JAMA, 94*:1136, 1930.

Everts, William H.: The treatment of myasthenia gravis by the oral administration of prostigmin. *Bull Neurol Inst, 4*:523–530, 1935.

Fraser, D. C.: Myasthenia gravis in the dog. *J Neurol Neurosurg Psychiat, 33*:431–437, 1970.

Frenkel, M.: Treatment of myasthenia gravis by ovulatory suppression. *Arch Neurol (Chicago), 11*:613–617, 1964.

Gammon, George D.: Foreword, symposium on myasthenia gravis. *Amer J Med, 19*:655, 1955.

Glaser, Gilbert H.: Crises, precrises and drug resistance in myasthenia gravis. *Ann NY Acad Sci, 135*:335–345, 1966.

Goni, A. R.: *Myasthenia Gravis.* Baltimore, Williams & Wilkins Co., 1946.

Grinker, Roy R., Bucy, Paul C., and Sahs, Adolph L.: *Neurology,* 5th ed. Springfield, Charles C Thomas, 1960, pp. 1116–1121.

Grob, David, and Johns, Richard J.: Use of oximes in the treatment of intoxication by anticholinesterase compounds in normal subjects. *Amer J Med, 24*:497–511, 1958.

Grob, David, and Johns, Richard J.: Further studies on the mechanism of the defect in neuromuscular transmission in myasthenia gravis, with particular reference to the acetylocholine insensitive block. In *Myasthenia Gravis,* edited by Henry Viets. Springfield, Charles C Thomas, 1961, pp. 127.

Harvey, McGehee A.: *Textbook of Medicine.* Philadelphia, W. B. Saunders, 1967, pp. 1675.

Herrmann, Christian, Jr.: Myasthenia gravis. Brief guide to diagnosis and management. *Calif Med, 106*:275–281, 1967.

Josephson, E. M.: *The Thymus, Manganese and Myasthenia Gravis.* New York, Chedney Press, 1961.

Keane, James R., and Hoyt, William F.: Myasthenia (vertical) nystagmus. Verification by edrophonium tonography. *JAMA, 212*:1209–1210, 1970.

Kirschner, P. A., Osserman, Kermit E., and Kark, Allen, E.: Studies in myasthenia gravis transcervical total thymectomy. *JAMA, 209*:906–910, 1969.

Klein, J., and Osserman, Kermit E.: Studies in myasthenia gravis. *New Eng J Med, 271*:177–181, 1964.

Klenner, F. R.: Letter to the editor. *Tri-State Med J,* Oct. 1954.

Kornfeld, P., Samuels, Arthur J., Wolf, Robert L., and Osserman, Kermit E.: Metabolism of ^{14}C-labeled pyridostigmine in myasthenia gravis. Evidence for multiple metabolites. *Neurology, 20*:634–671, 1970.

Knott, H. S.: Crisis in myasthenia. *Med Clin N Amer, 53*:285–291, 1969.

Laurent, L. P. E.: Clinical observations on the use of prostigmin in the treatment of myasthenia gravis. *Brit Med J, 1*:463, 1935.

Laurent, L. P. E., and Walther, W. W.: The influence of large doses of potassium chloride on myasthenia gravis. *Lancet, 228*:1434, 1935.

MacKenzie, K. R., Martin, Maurice J., and Howard, Frank M., Jr.: Myasthenia gravis: Psychiatric concomitants. *Canad Med Ass J, 100*:988–991, 1969.

McQuillen, M. P.: Hazard from antibiotics in myasthenia gravis. *Ann Intern Med, 73*:487–488, 1970.

Middleton, William, Morgan, Dale D., and Moyers, Jack: Neostigmine therapy for apnea occurring after administration of neomycine. *JAMA, 165*:2186, 1957.

Milhorat, A. T.: Choline-esterase activity of blood serum in disease. *J Clin Invest, 17*:649–657, 1938.

Milhorat, A. T., and Wolff, H. G.: Studies in diseases of muscle. III Metabolism of creatine and creatinine in myasthenia gravis including study of the excretion of nucleosides and nucleotides. *Arch Neurol Psychiat, 39*:354–372, 1938.

Namba, Tatsuji, Brown, Stuart C., and Grob, David: Neonatal myasthenia gravis: Report of two cases with review of the literature. *Pediatrics, 45*:488–504, 1970.

Nastuk, W. L., and Plescia, O. J.: Current status of research on myasthenia gravis. *Ann NY Acad Sci, 135*:664–678, 1966.

Nastuk, W. L., Strauss, A. J., and Osserman, Kermit E.: Search for a neuromuscular blocking agent in the blood of patients with myasthenia gravis. *Amer J Med, 26*:394–409, 1959.

Oosterhius, H. J.: Studies in myasthenia gravis: A clinical study of 180 patients. *J Neurol Sci, 1*:512–546, 1964.

Osserman, Kermit E.: *Myasthenia Gravis.* New York, Grune & Stratton, 1958.

Osserman, Kermit E.: Myasthenia gravis in *Current Therapy.* Philadelphia, London, Toronto, W. B. Saunders, 1971, pp. 630–638.

Osserman, Kermit E., and Genkins, Gabriel: Critical reappraisal of the use of edrophonium (tensilon) chloride tests in myasthenia gravis and significance of clinical classification. *Ann NY Acad Sci, 135*:312–326, 1966.

Osserman, Kermit E., and Shapiro, Elaine E.: Nursing care in myasthenia gravis. *Nursing World, 130*:6, 1956.

Osserman, Kermit E., and Teng, Paul: Studies in myasthenia gravis: A rapid diagnostic test. *JAMA, 160*:153–155, 1956.

Parets, Albert D.: Emotional reactions to chronic physical illness. *Med Clin N Amer 51*:1399, 1967.

Perlo, Vincent P., Poskanzer, David C., Schwab, Robert S. Viets, Henry R., Osserman, Kermit E., and Genkins, Gabriel: Myasthenia gravis: Evaluation of treatment in 1,355 patients. *Neurology, 16*:431–439, 1966.

Perlow, Samuel: Prostigmin in the treatment of peripheral circulatory disturbances. *JAMA, 114*:1991, 1940.

Phillips, Theodore: The Role of radiation therapy in myasthenia gravis. *Calif Med, 4*:106, 1967.

Ravin, H. A., Zacks, S. I., and Seligman, A. M.: Histochemical localization of acetylcholinesterase in nervous tissue. *J Pharmacol Exp Ther, 107*:37, 1953.

Rigotti, S., and Schergna, E.: A new drug for symptomatic treatment of myasthenia gravis: Mestinon. *JAMA, 156*:922, 1954.

Roberts, H. J.: *Difficult Diagnosis.* Philadelphia, W. B. Saunders, 1958, pp. 369–372.

Rose, Noel R., and Taylor, D. M.: The autoimmune diseases. *Med Clin N Amer, 49*:1675–1716, 1965.

Rowland, Lewis P.: Prostigmin-responsiveness and the diagnosis of myasthenia gravis. *Neurology, 5*:612–624, 1955.

Rowland Lewis P., Korengold, Marvin, Jaffe, Israeli, Berg, Leonard, and Shy, G. Milton: Prostigmine-induced muscle weakness in myasthenia gravis patients. *Neurology, 5*:89–99, 1955.

Rowland, Lewis P.: Myasthenia gravis in *Current Therapy.* Philadelphia, London, Toronto, W. B. Saunders, 1970, pp. 650–655.

Rowland, L. P., Osserman, Elliott F., Scharfman, William B., Balsom, Richard F., and Ball, Stanley: Myasthenia gravis with a mycloma-type gamma G (lgG) immunoglobulin abnormality. *Amer J Med, 46*:599–605, 1969.

Schulman, S., Rider, J. A., and Richter, R. B.: OMPA in myasthenia gravis. *JAMA, 152*:1707, 1953.

Schwab, Robert S., and Timberlake, William H.: Pyridostigmin (mestinon) in the treatment of myasthenia gravis. *New Eng J Med, 251*:271–272, 1954.

Schwab, Robert S., Marshall, Clarke K., and Timberlake, William: WIN 8077 (mysuran) in the treatment of myasthenia gravis. *JAMA, 158*:625, 1955.

Schwab, Robert S.: Problems in the diagnosis and treatment of myasthenia gravis. *Med Clin N Amer 47*:1511, 1963.

Schwartz, Herbert: Urecholine in myasthenia gravis. *Canad Med Ass J,* 72:346–351, 1955.

Slaughter, Donald, and Munsell, Donald: Some new aspects of morphine action; effects on pain. *J. Pharmacol,* 88:104, 1940.

Soskin, Samuel, Wachtel, Hans, and Hechter, Oscar: The treatment of delayed menstruation with prostigmin. *JAMA, 114:*2090, 1940.

Summers, J. S.: Myasthenia gravis. *J Missouri State Med Ass, 179:*82, 1933.

Teng, Paul, and Osserman, Kermit E.: Studies in myasthenia gravis: Neonatal and juvenile types. *J Mt Sinai Hosp, 23:*711–727, 1956.

Tether, J. E.: Mestinon in myasthenia gravis. Preliminary report, *Dis Nerv Syst, 15:*227, 1954.

Thesleff, S.: Neuromuscular block caused by acetylcholine. *Nature, 175:* 594–595, 1955.

Taquini, Alberto C., Cooke, W. Trever, and Schwab, Robert S.: Observations in cardiovascular system in myasthenia gravis. *Amer Heart J, 20:* 611, 1940.

Van de Velde, R. L., and Friedman, Nathan B.: Thymicmyoid cells and myasthenia gravis. *Amer J Path, 59:*347–368, 1970.

Viets, Henry R., and Mitchell, R. S.: Prostigmin in the diagnosis of myasthenia gravis. *New Eng J Med, 213:*1280, 1935.

Walker, M. B.: Case showing effect of prostigmin on myasthenia gravis. *Proc Roy Soc Med, 28:*759, 1935.

Walker, M. B.: Treatment of myasthenia gravis with physostigmine. *Lancet,* 1:1200–1201, 1934.

Yoel, J., and Alurralde, A.: The carotid sinus and myasthenia gravis. *JAMA, 165:*2010, 1957.

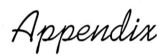

FORMS OF MYASTHENIA GRAVIS

1. Juvenile
    a. Myasthenic mother transfers symptoms to baby. Shows up at birth then disappears.
    b. Symptoms develop during childhood, generally around eight or nine years of age. Affects both sides equally. Mother not a myasthenic but frequently there are cases in the family.
2. Adult
    a. Mild form which can affect a single group of muscles, manifested in a drooping eyelid or double vision in one eye only.
    b. Severe form affects the total body. It may include tumor on thymus or muscle atrophy.

DEVELOPMENT OF THE DISEASE

1672—First paper written on M. G. by Thomas Willis, an Englishman. Described the disease. No treatment given.

1879—First fully reported accounts of patients with M. G. by Erb.

1927—Up to this time only 300 cases reported. Treatment restricted to rest, large doses of strychnine, sometimes arsenic, thyroid extract, parathyroid preparations, calcium and thorium.

1930—Ephedrine sulphate first used by Dr. Harriet Edgeworth.

1934—Glycine used by McGuire.

1935—Prostigmin introduced by Dr. Mary Walker.
Oral Prostigmin introduced by Dr. William H. Everts.
Prostigmin used as a diagnostic test by Viets and Schwab.
Insulin used as treatment for M. G. by Pitfield.
Anterior pituitary extract used by Simon.
Use of potassium chloride introduced by Laurent.
Milhorat reported use of liver arginase.

1936—Radiology first used on thymus of myasthenic patient by Everts.

1939—Thymectomy first used by Blalock.

1948—Use of hexaethyltetraphosphate reported by Westerberg and Lures.
ACTH first used.

1949—Effects of TEPP on treatment of M. G. noted by Grob and Harvey.

1951—Octamethylpyrophosphoramide developed. Rider, Schulman, Richter, Moeller, DeBois.
Tensilon developed by Westerberg, Magee, Shiderman.

1952—Tensilon used as diagnostic test by Osserman, Kaplan.

1954—Mestinon reported by Osserman.

1955—Mytelase reported by Schwab.
Urecholine reported by Schwartz.

1956—Mysuran introduced by Westerberg.

1957—Carotid sinus operation for M. G. introduced by Alurralde.

THEORIES OF CAUSES

1. Competitive-type block which inhibits motor end-plate depolarizing action of acetylcholine released from motor nerve endings.

2. Dysfunction of endocrine system, either adrenals or para-thyroid, which causes disturbances in sympathetic nervous system causing impaired blood supply to muscle.
3. Failure of thymus gland to shrink at puberty or a tumor on the thymus.
4. Breakdown in protein enzyme metabolism.
5. Bacteria between muscle fibers give off toxins which cause muscle fatigue.
6. An autoimmunity disease in which the body reacts to ab-normal cells by building antibodies and retains them at junction of muscles and nerves.

RANGE OF SYMPTOMS OF THE DISEASE

1. Drooping eyelid in one or both eyes.
2. Fatigue upon slightest motion.
3. Heaviness in legs.
4. Double vision.
5. Difficulty in chewing or swallowing.
6. Sagging jaws.
7. Masked facial expression.
8. Voice weakness. Voice becomes inaudible.
9. Weakness of cardiac muscles which may cause palpita-tions or abnormally rapid heart action.
10. Weakness in arms and legs.
11. Neck muscles may be so weak it is difficult to hold head erect.
12. Feel best in morning, weaken as day progresses.
13. Weakness improves following rest.

SELECTED READINGS

This list presents only a few suggested books and magazines which might prove helpful. It has not been selected as representative of the best in each area. The purpose of the list is to provide a starting point to stimulate your exploration of other resources.

Adults

Brande, Dorothea: *Wake Up and Live.* New York, Cornerstone Library, 1968. (Paperback)

This book will help you reach goals and achieve success through profitable thinking, new personal standards of energy conservation, new speech habits, creative self-discipline and positive action.

Stout, Ruth: *If You Would Be Happy.* New York, Cornerstone Library, 1969. (Paperback)

Author gives simple things to correct muddled thinking, stops you from reaching for the unreachable and tells how to find within yourself the essential ingredients for greater enjoyment and contentment. She helps you to achieve true happiness and make it last in spite of adversity and loss.

Entertainment

Depew, Arthur M.: *The Cokesbury Game Book.* Nashville, Abingdon Press, 1959.

Eisenberg, Helen and Larry: *The Omnibus of Fun.* New York, Association Press, 1956.

Ickis, Marguerite: *Pastimes for the Patient.* New York, American Book Company, 1966.

Masters, Robert V.: *The Family Game Book.* New York, Doubleday, 1967.

Tedford, Jack: *The Giant Book of Family Fun and Games.* New York, Watts, 1958.

Thomsen, Robert: *Games, Anyone?* New York, Doubleday, 1968. (Paperback)

Wood, Clement and Goddard, Gloria (Eds.): *The Complete Book of Games.* New York, Doubleday, 1938.

Health

Books

Hofmann, Ruth B.: *How to Build Special Furniture and Equipment for Handicapped Children.* Springfield, Charles C Thomas, 1970.

Jacobson, Edmund, M.D.: *You Must Relax,* 4th ed. New York, McGraw, 1957.

> A book explaining methods successfully used in Dr. Jacobson's clinics in Chicago and New York which teach people the secret of "taking it easy" and yet getting one's daily work done.

Ruslink, Doris: *Family Health and Home Nursing.* New York, Macmillan, 1963.

> Suggestions for caring for the patient with ease and understanding his needs.

Magazines

Accent on Living, 802 Reinthaler, Bloomington, Ill. Editor: Raymond C. Cheever.

> Rehabilitation success stories and news of new ideas and products developed to make living easier for people with disabilities. (Quarterly—$2.00, 50¢ per copy).

Children's Telescope, The. Handicapped Children's Home Service, 105 W. 55th Street, New York 19, N. Y.

Family Health. Family Health Magazine, Inc., 1271 Avenue of the Americas, New York, N. Y. 10010. Editor: Wm. H. White.

> Current news on health care in language for layman.

Fitness for Living. Rodale Press, Inc., 33 E. Minor St., Emmaus, Pa. 18049. Editor: John Haberern

> Covers all areas of physical fitness designed to interest the general public. Bimonthly—$3.00 a year.

Today's Health. American Medical Association, 535 N. Dearborn St., Chicago, Ill. 60610. Editor: Elliott H. McCleary.

> Medical and scientifically correct articles written for the lay person. $4.00 a year, 50¢ a copy.

Health Care. P. O. Box 251, Madison Square Station, New York, N. Y. 10010. Editor: Jessyca Russell Gaver.

Nutrition, exercise, family, home care for invalids and nursing homes. 60¢ a copy.

Hobbies

Hall, H. J., and Knox, M. M.: *Handicrafts for the Handicapped.* New York, Dodd.

Hobbies. Lightner Publishing Corp., 1006 S. Michigan Ave., Chicago, Illinois 60605. $4.00 a year; 50¢ a copy.

Authentic articles and stories about everything old, historic or antique.

Hobbies to Enjoy. Hobbies to Enjoy, Inc., 5038 Winona Ave., St. Louis, Mo. 63169. Editor: Al Wick.

Coins, stamps, match covers, post-covers, seashells, minerals, travel, Hobby Club news. Quarterly—$2.00.

Hobby Times and Bookworm. Box 76, Rockport, Maine 04856. Editor: Jacqueline Steele. $2.50 a year; 35¢ a copy.

Home Workshop. Science and Mechanics Publishing Co., 229 Park Ave. S., New York, N. Y. 10003. 75¢ per copy.

The National Hobbyist. National Hobby Institute, Cape Coral Gardens, Cape Coral, Fla., 22904.

1001 How-to-Ideas. Science and Mechanics Publishing Co., 505 Park Ave. S., New York, N. Y. 10022.

Workbasket. Modern Handcraft, Inc., 4251 Penn Ave., Kansas City, Mo., 64111. Editor: Mary Ida Sullivan.

Patterns and directions to knit, tat, crochet, recipes, crafts and hobbies, garden information, money-making opportunities. Quarterly—25¢ per copy. $1.00 per year.

Workbench. Modern Handcraft, Inc., 4251 Penn Ave., Kansas City, Mo. 64111. Editor: Jay W. Hedden.

Tested plans for home workshop projects, guidance on home remodeling, refinishing, sources of tools and supplies. Bimonthly—$2.00, 35¢ a copy.

Nutrition

Better Homes and Gardens Nutrition for Your Family. New York, Meredith, 1961.

A guide book for better family nutrition.

Bogert, Jean L.: *Nutrition and Physical Fitness*, 8th ed. Philadelphia, Saunders, 1966.

A textbook in nontechnical language about the facts of foods.

Cooper, Lenna F., and Mitchell, Helen S.: *Cooper's Nutrition in Health and Disease*, 15th ed. Philadelphia, Lippincott, 1968.

A handbook for nurses and homemakers. It gives the principles of nutrition and has chapters on diet in disease and instructions for cooking for the sick and convalescent.

Davis, Adelle: *Let's Eat Right to Keep Fit.* New York, Harcourt, Brace & World, 1954. (Paperback by Signet, 1970.)

A world famous nutritionist's best-selling guide to physical and emotional well-being through proper diet. Other books by the same author: *Let's Cook It Right* (a cookbook) (Rev. ed. 1962) *Let's Have Healthy Children* (Rev. 1959).

Davis, Adelle: *Let's Get Well.* New York, Harcourt, Brace & World, 1965.

A very readable explanation of the part various food elements play in keeping us well, written by a noted nutritionist.

Leverton, Ruth M.: *Food Becomes You.* Iowa State University Press, 1965. (Paperback by Dolphin Doubleday.)

Clear, concise information on nutrition by specialist in field.

Williams, Roger J.: *Nutrition in a Nutshell.* New York, Doubleday, 1962.

A noted biochemist examines our food needs and how we can meet them sensibly.

Personal Understanding and Development

Children

Gesell, Arnold, and Ilg, Frances L.: *Child Development.* New York, Harper & Row, 1949.

A study of the growth and development of children.

Reeves, Katherine: *Children—Their Ways and Wants.* Darien (Conn.), Educational Publishing Corp., 1959.

With clarity, humor and compassion, the author shows why one child must rebel, why another is shy, and another a bully. Explains what learning is, explores the child's fears and anxieties.

Strang, Ruth: *Helping Your Child Develop His Potentialties.* New York, Dutton, 1965.

Ways to promote growth in children from infancy through adolescence.

Adolescents

Baruch, Dorothy: *How to Live With Your Teenager.* New York, McGraw, 1953.

Suggested approaches to some of the situations that arise between parents and their adolescent children. Also by author: *New Ways in Discipline.*

Daly, Sheila John: *Personality Plus.* New York, Dodd, 1964.

Discusses school and personal life with hints on how to get along with parents, secure a date, overcome shyness, and plan a career.

Duvall, Evelyn M.: *Todays Teen-Agers.* New York, Association Press, 1966.

A parent's guide to everyday problems of boys and girls: dating, clothes, social life, dropout, sex, and marriage.

Johnson, Eric W.: *How to Live Through Junior High*. Philadelphia, Lippincott, 1959.

> Practical guide to dealing with and living with children experiencing the confusing emotions and problems of early adolescence.

Menninger, William C.: *How To Be A Successful Teenager*. New York, Sterling, 1966.

> Informal and informative handbook directed to school, religious counselors, youth leaders, parents and students themselves.

Sugarman, D. L., and Hochstein, R.: *Seventeen's Guide to Knowing Yourself*. New York, Macmillan, 1968.

> A guide to self-discovery and maturity for high school girls. Advice on emotion and social life. How to handle anger and fear, minimize friction with parents, going slow in love, sex and early marriage.

Adults

Adler, Alfred: *What Life Should Mean to You*. Paperback by Putnam, 1959.

Adolph, Paul: *Release from Tension*. Paperback by Moody, 1959.

Cooper, Joseph D.: *How to Get More Done in Less Time*. New York, Doubleday, 1962.

Fink, David H.: *For People Under Pressure*. New York, Simon & Schuster, 1956.

> A neuropsychiatrist attempts to answer questions patients ask such as understanding self, building self-confidence, expressing yourself, winning loyal friends, and making profitable decisions.

Kutscher, Austin H.: *But Not to Lose*. New York, Fell, 1959.

> A book of comfort for those bereaved. A help in accepting and resolving grief and in resuming a productive life.

Liebman, Joshua, L.: *Hope for Man*. New York, Simon & Schuster, 1966.

An optimistic and philosophical guide to self-fulfillment. Also by same author: *Peace of Mind* (New York, Simon & Schuster, 1965 paperback). (Large-typed 1969, Clarion, S&S.)

Mander, A. E.: *Trying to Understand People:* Psychology for Everyday Use. New York, Taplinger, 1967. (Paperback)
May, Rollo: *Man's Search for Himself.* New York, Norton, 1953. (Also in paperback by Signet.)

A psychologist examines the nature of modern man's insecurities and offers suggestions for better understanding of self and needs—written for laymen. Also by author: *Love and Will,* a more profound discussion of man's struggle in today's society.

Shacter, Helen: *Understanding Ourselves.* New York, McKnight, 1959. Paperback.

To help the individual understand people better and to gain insight into reasons why people behave as they do.

Psychology

McDonald, Eugene T.: *Understanding Those Feelings.* Pittsburgh (Pa.) Stanwix House, Inc., 1962.

A guide for parents of handicapped children and for everyone who counsels them.

Retirement

Blanchard, Fessenden S.: *Make the Most of Your Retirement.* New York, Doubleday, 1963.

Where to go, what to do and how much it costs.

Buckley, Jos. C.: *The Retirement Handbook.* New York, Harper & Row, 1962.

A complete guide to planning your future.

Myasthenia Gravis

Myasthenia Gravis: A Handbook for Patients.

A 12 page booklet which provides the answers to most frequently asked questions. Available free from M. G. Foundation and chapter offices.

Myasthenia Gravis: A Manual for the Physician.

A 28 page booklet to aid the practicing physician in the recognition, management and understanding of myasthenia gravis. Available free for professional use from the M. G. Foundation and chapter offices.

M. G. Fact Sheet.

A government pamphlet free from the National Institute of Neurological Diseases and Stroke, Bldg. 36, Rm. 4D—04, Bethesda, Md. 20014.

Miscellaneous

Job Wanted.

Pamphlet dealing with rehabilitation and job-finding services and small business opportunities. Presidents Committee and National Multiple Sclerosis Society, Washington, D.C. 20210.

Guide to the National Parks and Monuments for Handicapped Tourists.

President's Committee and the Veteran's Employment Service of the U. S. Department of Labor Manpower Administration, Washington, D. C. 20210.

Fashion-Able Catalog.

Fashions and aids for the handicapped. Rocky Hill, New Jersey 08553.

Index

$\diamondsuit\diamond\diamondsuit\diamond\diamondsuit\diamond\diamondsuit\diamond\diamondsuit\diamond\diamondsuit\diamond\diamondsuit\diamond\diamondsuit\diamond\diamondsuit\diamond\diamondsuit\diamond\diamondsuit\diamond\diamondsuit\diamond\diamondsuit\diamond\diamondsuit\diamond\diamondsuit\diamond\diamondsuit\diamond\diamondsuit\diamond\diamondsuit$